123 Healthy Paleo Diet Recipes

By

Rebecca Publishing

Disclaimer

All the material contained in this book is provided for informational and educational purposes only. No responsibility can be taken for any outcomes resulting from the use of this material.

While every attempt has been made to provide information that is both accurate and effective, the author does not assume any responsibility for the accuracy or use/misuse of this information.

About the author!

I have been studying healthy way of eating from leading nutritionist in Europe and I have a lot of useful information on this topic. I have lost more than 20 kilos so I can provide you with a lot of practical tips on this matter.

My story is also very bright, after giving birth to a child; I have gained a lot of extra weight. It was simply impossible to look into the mirror, but I decided to do my best to return to my previous shape. I have tried swimming, jogging, different diets like Dukan, Sugar Free Diet, Kremlyovskaya Diet etc. These diets forced me to starving and nothing more. I saw and fell the best result after following the Paleo Diet. This diet helped me to loose ALL my extra weight this is more than 20 kilos/44 pounds and I feel myself much healthier now! So, Let's start my explanation of what is it – paleo diet and the main aspects of it.

The History of Paleo Diet

I would like to tell you some words about the history of the Paleo Diet. This diet was developed and presented in the 1970s by the doctor, actually gastroenterologist. The name of this person is Walter Voegtlin. The main suggestion of him was to eat like our forefathers and become healthier, stronger and lean in such a way. What is more he claimed that this diet can reduce a lot of health problems such as diabetes, obesity and even Crohn`s disease. . It helps you to better your mental health. This diet is also a great way to make your face look better without spots and acne. What is more paleo diet makes a positive affect to your immune system as well as your digestion system. To crown it all the paleo diet can help you to minimize your blood pressure and better your sleep.

Mr Walter Voegtlin claimed, the main principles of this diet is to eat everything what our Paleolithic men consumed. These are mainly the following products: meats and fish (because it was easy to hunt for) also nuts, seeds, different fruits and vegetable. Everything is simple. Now I would like to proceed to the first chapter where. I am going to list more than 100 recipes of Healthy Paleo Dishes.

The contents

BREAKFAST, LUNCH AND DINNER RECIPES

1. Flax Almond Meal Banana Muffins with Dark Chocolate

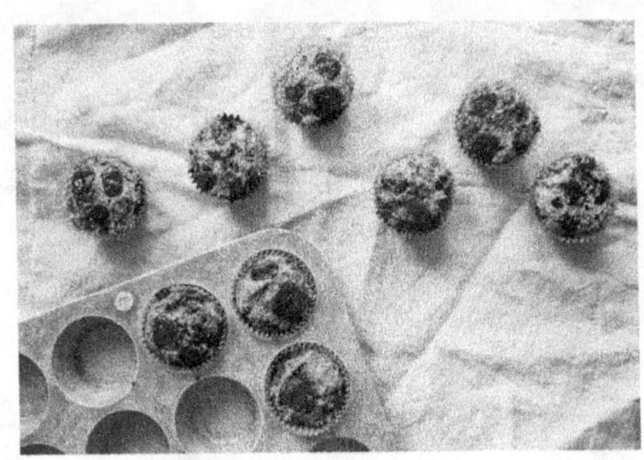

INGREDIENTS (for 10 muffins)
Almond meal – 155 g
Flaxseed meal – 35 g
Baking powder – 5 g
Cinnamon – 2,5 g
Bananas – 2 pcs
Egg – 1 piece
Coconut oil – 5 ml
Apple cider vinegar – 5 ml
Vanilla extract – 5 g
Unsweetened almond milk – 10 ml
Dark chocolate – 70 gr (72%)
A pinch of salt

INSTRUCTIONS
1. First of all, prepare the oven. Turn it on and heat to 190 C.
2. Take a medium sized bowl and combine dry ingredients. Whisk well. Set aside.
3. Mash bananas in a large separate bowl. Add there slightly beaten egg, coconut oil, vanilla, apple cider vinegar and almond milk. Mix until smooth.
4. Chop dark chocolate. Combine mixed dry ingredients and banana mousse. Add some chocolate chunks. Stir carefully. Your muffin batter is ready.
5. Take muffin cups, grease them with oil and fill 3/4 of the way full.
6. Bake in preheated oven for 20-25 minutes.
7. Sprinkle each muffin with grated chocolate on top.
<u>Nutritional values (for 1 muffin without chocolate)</u>

Carbs - 9.9 g, fiber - 3.6 g, protein - 6.3 g, fat - 13.4 g, energy – 180 kcal
<u>Nutrition values (for 1 muffin with chocolate)</u>Carbs - 13 g, fiber – 4.2 g, protein - 6.8 g, fat - 16.7g, energy – 218 kcal

2. *Chicken Samosa Hash (breakfast)*

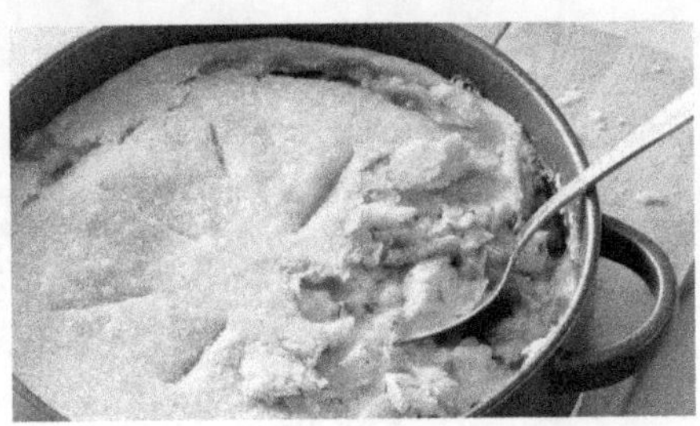

INGREDIENTS (for 4 servings)
Eggs – 8 pcs
Ground chicken – 450 gr
Coconut oil – 60 ml
White vinegar – 10 ml
Onion – 1 piece
Garlic bulbets – 2 pcs,
Jalapenos – 2 pcs
Rutabaga – 1 piece
Fresh spinach – 200 gr
Red chili powder – 10 gr
Cumin – 10 gr
Cinnamon – 2,5 gr
Ground ginger – 10 gr
Curry powder – 34 gr+25 gr
Salt and ground black pepper
Fresh cilantro – one handful

INSTRUCTIONS
1. Prepare vegetables and greens. Peel and mince 2-3 garlic bulbets, dice jalapenos, onion and rutabaga, chop spinach and fresh cilantro.
2. Take a skillet and melt coconut oil. Add cumin, cinnamon, ginger, curry and red chili powder. Cook for one minute. Don't forget to stir constantly. Add prepared onion, garlic and jalapenos. Sauté for one-two minutes.
3. Now add ground chicken. Stir it carefully to break into small pieces. Now its time for diced rutabaga. Put it in the skillet, cover the pan. Let simmer for ten minutes. After 10 minutes, add chopped spinach.
4. Season this fragrant mixture with salt and pepper to taste. Remove the skillet from heat.
5. Meanwhile, take a saucepan and pour some water in it. Bring to a boil and add some salt and 10 ml of white vinegar. Then carefully poach the eggs. Switch of the heat, cover the saucepan and wait for 5 minutes, until eggs will be ready.
6. Turn the hash and poached eggs on the plate. Serve with chopped fresh cilantro.

Nutritional values (per 1 serving)
Carbs - 12 g, protein - 31 g, fat - 46 g, energy – 511 kcal

3. Shrimp Fried Cauliflower "Rice" (Lunch)

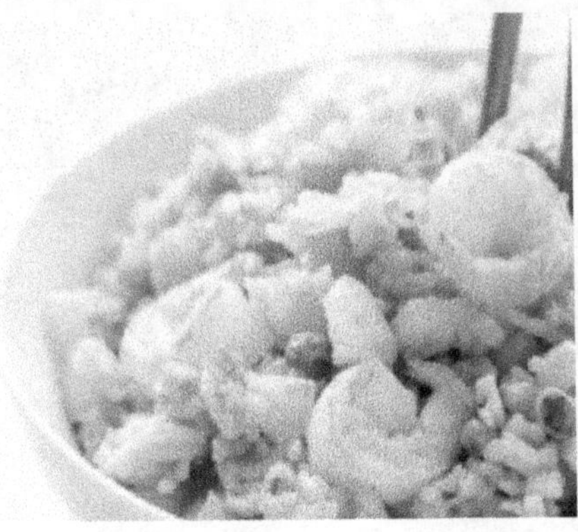

INGREDIENTS (for 4 servings)
Cauliflower - 2 heads
Duck or bacon fat – 30 gr
Egg – 1 piece
Shallots – 30-40 gr
Red bell pepper – 1 piece
Green bell pepper – 1 piece
Carrot – 1 piece
Shrimp – 450 gr
Soy sauce – 45 ml
Fish sauce – 3 drops
Sesame oil (toasted) – 7 ml
Green onion – 1/4
Salt and pepper

INSTRUCTIONS
1. Make preparations. Wash vegetables and dry with paper towel. Peel carrot and dice it, chop red and green bell pepper, dice shallots. Cut cauliflower heads into big pieces. Use ricer to make puree (instead of ricer you may use grater to grate cauliflower). Peel shrimps.
2. Melt fat in the pan and add chopped peppers, diced shallots and carrot. Fry on medium fire for 3–4 minutes.
3. Now add peeled shrimps to vegetables and stir. Pour liquid ingredients: soy sauce, fish sauce and sesame oil.
4. When the shrimps are pink and fully cooked, beat the egg and whisk with the fork.
5. Mix riced cauliflower with green onion and pour in the pan. Add salt and pepper to taste, and cook until the cauliflower is ready.

6. Serve warm!
Nutritional values (per 1 serving)
Carbs - 17 g, protein - 31 g, fat - 8 g, energy – 267 kcal

4. Sweet & Spicy Cashews

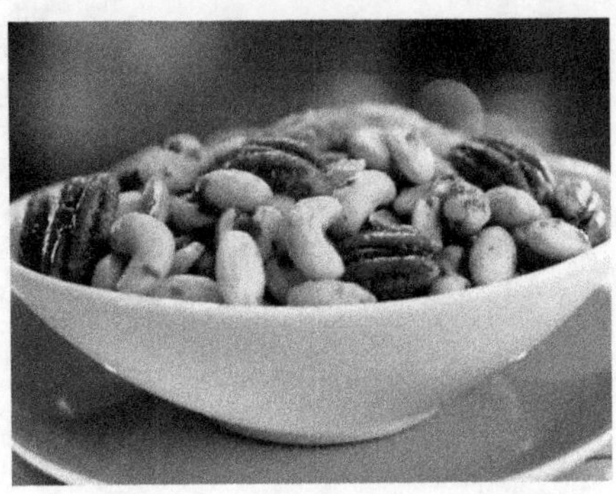

INGREDIENTS (for 8 servings)
Honey – 85 gr
Raw cashews – 170 g
Coconut sugar – 50 gr
Coconut oil – 10 gr
Smoked paprika – 2,5 gr
Cayenne pepper – 1,5+1 gr
Salt 1,5 gr
Pinch of sea salt

INSTRUCTIONS
1. Preheat the oven to 190°C, line the baking sheet with pergament paper.
2. Combine 1 gr of paprika, 1,5 gr of cayenne pepper, and 1 gr of salt. Melt coconut oil and mix it with honey, add dry spices. Whisk carefully. Add raw cashews, and stir. Cashews should be fully coated with this honey-spiced mixture. Spread coated cashews over the baking sheet.
3. Combine remaining paprika, cayenne, and salt. Dust the cashews.
4. Bake cashews for 15 minutes, stirring constantly to ensure they don't burn.
5. Remove cashews. Let cool and enjoy!
Nutritional values (per 1 serving)
Carbs - 23 g, protein - 5 g, fat - 17 g, energy – 250 kcal

5. Sweet Potato Pasta with Prosciutto, Goat Cheese & Figs

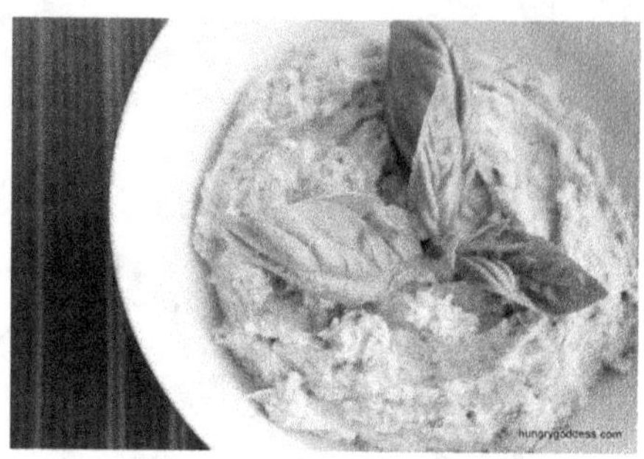

INGREDIENTS (for 4 servings)

Sweet potato – 2 pcs
Crumbled goat cheese – 15 gr
Dried figs – 15 pcs
Prosciutto – 115 gr
Slivered almonds – 1 cup
Olive oil – 7 ml
Water – 30 ml
Sea salt – 2,5 gr

INSTRUCTIONS
1. Take sweet potatoes, peel them, chop the ends off and make long strands with spiralizer
2. Heat the skillet with olive oil and put sweet potato strands to the pan, salt to taste. Cook 5-7 min until tender. Remove the pan and turn noodles on the plate.
3. Cut prosciutto into 1-inch sticks and fry in the same skillet for 3 minutes, stirring constantly.
4. Add sliced into rounds figs and almonds, fry for 3 minutes more until figs are browned. Add half of crumbled goat cheese and cook until cheese is started melting.
5. Add 30 ml of water and transfer the sweet potato noodles again in the pan. Mix thoroughly.
6. Turn the noodles on the dish and drizzle with remaining crumbled goat cheese.
7. Your tasty Sweet Potato Pasta with Prosciutto, Goat Cheese and Figs is ready!
Nutritional values (per 1 serving)
Carbs - 59 g, protein - 22 g, fat - 26 g, energy – 534 kcal

6. Honey Bunches of Paleo Cereal

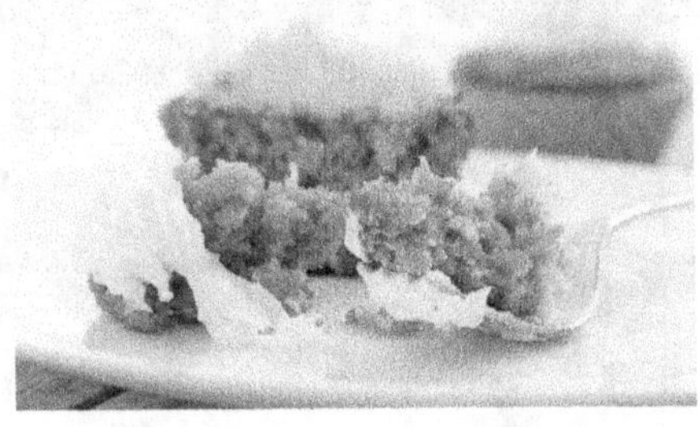

INGREDIENTS (for 8 servings)
Unsalted sunflower seeds – 85 gr
Unsweetened coconut flakes – 1 cup
Unsalted walnut pieces – 85 gr
Dried unsweetened cherries – 21 gr
Raw almond butter – 50 gr
Raw honey – 85 gr
Coconut flour – 32 gr
Coconut oil

INSTRUCTIONS
1. Preheat the oven to 175 C. Grease your baking sheet with coconut oil.
2. Combine all ingredients in a bowl and blend well. Press mixture into greased baking sheet.
3. Bake until browned for 15-20 minutes. Let cool. Crumble into container.
4. Serve with unsweetened coconut milk (if you like)
5. Enjoy!
Nutritional values (per 1 serving)
Carbs - 20 g, protein - 6 g, fat – 24 g, energy – 308 kcal

7. Baked Breakfast Casserole with Apples and Raisins

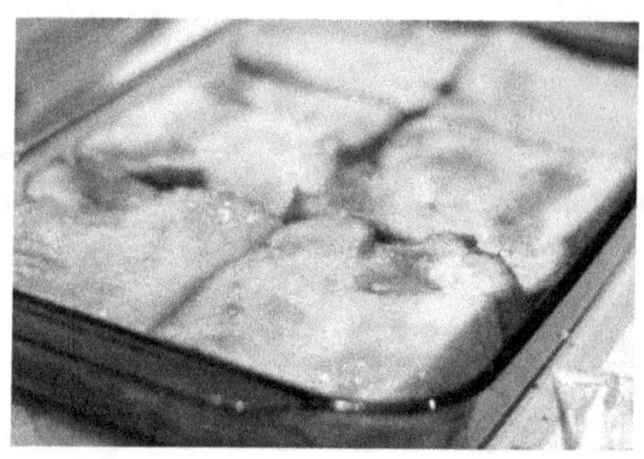

INGREDIENTS (for 6 servings)
Cooked spaghetti squash flesh – 4 cups
Banana – 1 piece
Apple – 1 piece
Ground cinnamon – 7,5 gr
Ground mace – 1,5 g
Applesauce – 120 ml
Avocado oil – 60 ml
Raisins – 100 gr
Gelatin powder – 50 gr
Tapioca starch – 50 gr
Baking soda – 12 gr
Cream of tartar – 5 gr
Sea salt
Vanilla extract

INSTRUCTIONS
1. Make preparations: combine cooked spaghetti squash flesh, raisins, ground mace, mashed banana, diced apple, ground cinnamon, applesauce, vanilla extract, avocado oil and sea salt in a large bowl. Put in the refrigerator overnight .
2. Take another bowl and combine tapioca starch, gelatin powder and baking soda. Mix well and add 5 gr of cream of tartar.
3. The next day: Preheat your oven to 177C. Remove cold squash mixture from the fridge. Grease your glass casserole dish.
4. Mix dry ingredients with cold squash mixture and stir well. Fill greased casserole dish with prepared mixture .
5. Cover the dish with foil and bake for one hour.
6. Serve warm or cold!

Nutritional values (per 1 serving)
Carbs - 31 g, protein – 3 g, fat – 2 g, energy – 141 kcal

8. Baked Breakfast Quinoa with Dates & Banana

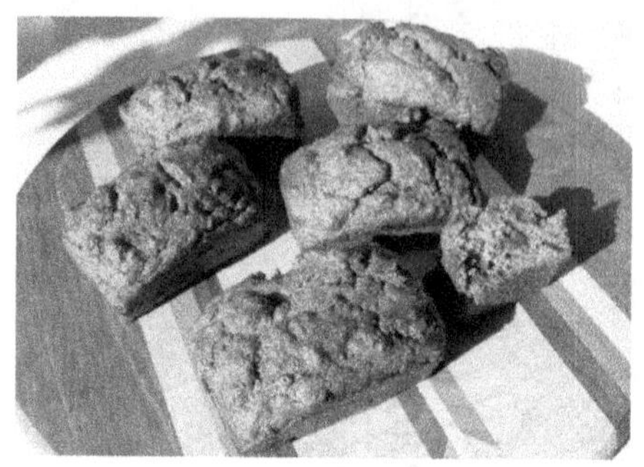

INGREDIENTS (for 6 servings)
<u>For the Quinoa:</u>
Uncooked quinoa – 1 cup
Unsweetened vanilla almond milk – 240 ml
Unsweetened regular almond milk – 240 ml
Honey – 120 gr
Cinnamon – 2,5 gr
Egg – 2 pcs
Water – 120 ml
Salt
<u>For the date filling:</u>
Dates – 1 cup   roughly chopped
Water – 240 ml
Coconut sugar – 25 gr
For the streusel:
Banana – 1 piece
Coconut oil - 25 g+5 gr
Coconut sugar – 50 gr
Almond flour – 32 gr
Slivered almonds – ¼ cup
Cinnamon – 1 gr

INSTRUCTIONS
1. Make preparations: preheat the oven to 175C, take a pie dish and grease it with oil. Also line the bottom of your dish with oil-paper. Set aside for some time.

2. Its time to cook the quinoa: look at the list of ingredients. Take a large pot and pour unsweetened vanilla almond milk and unsweetened regular almond milk. Bring milks to a boil.

3. Stir in the raw quinoa, 120 gr of honey , 2,5 gr of cinnamon and add a dash of salt. Cover and put into the oven. Slack the fire and bake the quinoa until milk is absorbed and the quinoa is creamy(about 25-30 minutes).

4. Meanwhile, you may cook the date filling. First of all, wash dates and then chop them. Take a saucepan and put there chopped dates, 25 gr of coconut sugar and pour water. Make this mixture boil. Then reduce the heat and simmer 15 minutes until thick.

5. Directly after this, make date puree with a fork. Set it aside.

6. Its time to make the topping for quinoa: Take a bowl and combine 50 gr of coconut sugar, 32 gr of almond flour, ¼ cup of slivered almonds and a dash of cinnamon. Add coconut oil and mix until you get a uniform mass. Set aside.

7. After half an hour look at quinoa. It is ready! Transfer it into a larger bowl. Cracked a couple of eggs and pour remaining 120 ml of water. Mix thoroughly until soupy consistency.

8. Divide quinoa into two parts. Pour the first half into the prepared greased pie dish. Using a spoon spread date filling evenly over top of the quinoa . Pour the second half of quinoa over the date filling.

9. Slice bananas and cover the quinoa. At last, sprinkle the streusel topping to cover banana slices.

10. Bake 35 minutes. After 35 minutes, remove the quinoa from the oven. Let it cool and slice.

11. Devour!

Nutritional values (per 1 serving)

Carbs - 58 g, protein – 9 g, fat – 12 g, energy – 358 kcal

9. Easy Paleo Ham & Egg Cups

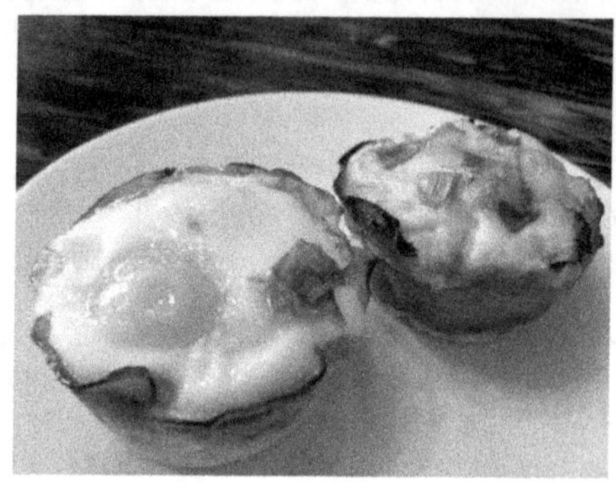

INGREDIENTS (for 6 servings)
Slices of ham – 6 pcs
Egg – 4 pcs
Full-cream coconut milk – 120 ml
Orange bell pepper - 1 piece
Red bell pepper – 1 piece
Yellow onion – 1 piece
Salt, pepper
Olive oil

INSTRUCTIONS
1. The oven must be preheated to 175 C.
2. Chop vegetables: onion and bell papers.
3. Take a saucepan, pour some oil and fry onions for 3-4 minutes, after add chopped peppers and fry for another 2 minutes. Set aside.
4. Next, stir up the eggs with the milk, salt and pepper to taste.
5. Grease baking cups with olive oil. Line each cup with ham slices and then fill with fried onion and peppers. Pour egg mixture.
6. Bake 20-30 minutes. Your Ham and Egg Cups are ready. Enjoy!
Nutritional values (per 1 serving)
Carbs - 3 g, protein – 10 g, fat – 11 g, energy – 150 kcal

10. Shrimp Tacos with Paleo Tortillas

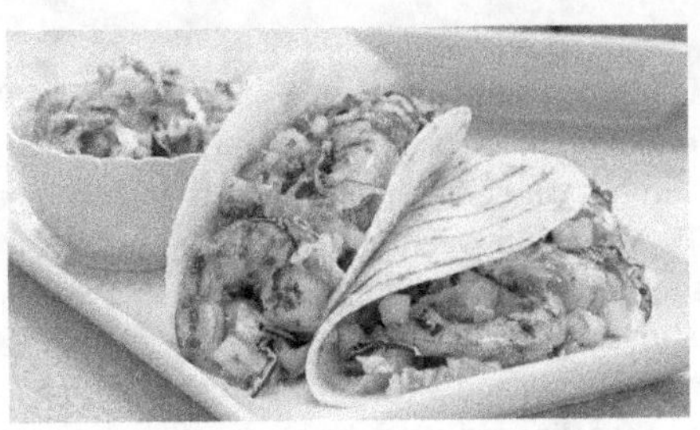

INGREDIENTS (for 5 servings)
<u>For bang bang sauce</u>
Homemade mayonnaise – 1/3 cup
Sweet chili sauce – 50 gr
Sriracha – 50 gr
<u>For sweet chili sauce</u>
White wine vinegar – 50 ml
Water – 30 ml
Honey – 40 gr
Garlic bulbet – 1 piece
Chili flakes – 5-7 gr
Minced ginger – 3 gr
Cayenne – 1 gr
Salt
<u>For tortillas</u>
Egg – 2 pcs   s
Water – 200 ml
Tapioca flour – 130 gr
Coconut flour – 130 gr
Salt – 2 gr
<u>For tacos</u>
Shrimp – 450 gr   , peeled
Tapioca flour – 50 gr
Honey – 15 gr
Coconut oil – 80 ml
Nappa cabbage – 1 cup
Red cabbage – ½ cup
Minced cilantro – ½ cup

Green onion – 2 pcs
Olive oil – 30 ml
 White wine vinegar – 15 ml. Salt

INSTRUCTIONS
Follow step-by-step instruction and cook unbelievable Shrimp Tacos with Paleo Tortillas.
1. First of all we should prepare sweet chili sauce because it is one of the components of bang bang sauce. To make this sweet chili sauce we need mince garlic and ginger and then combine them with all the rest ingredients. Mix well and pour in a saucepan. Turn on your oven and bring to a boil this fragrant mixture. Then slack the fire and simmer until thickened. Don't forget to stir constantly. Let cool. Sweet chili sauce is ready. To make bang bang sauce just add mayonnaise and Sriracha to chili sauce.
2. It's time to make tacos. In the first place shred nappa cabbage, red cabbage, mince cilantro and slice green onion. Take a bowl and combine these ingredients. Add two tablespoons of olive oil, one tablespoon of white wine vinegar, 15 gr of honey and a dash of salt. Set aside.
3. Now make the tortillas. In a separate bowl combine all ingredients for tortillas. Mix until smooth. Heat a pan, add olive oil. Pour the batter for one tortilla (one circle). Cook 1-2 minutes on the one side then turn and cook 1-2 minutes on the other side. When you finish you will have 6 soft, foldable and golden brown tortillas. Set aside.
4. Peel shrimps and toss with tapioca. Heat the pan and melt the coconut oil. Fry shrimps both sides until golden and crispy. Mix shrimps with Bang Bang sauce.
5. Put tacos on each tortilla and roll up. Top with shrimps in bang-bang sauce and drizzle with Sriracha.
Nutritional values (per serving)
Carbs - 46 g, protein – 25 g, fat – 30 g, energy – 555 kcal

11. Cuban Pork Lettuce Wraps (Lunch)

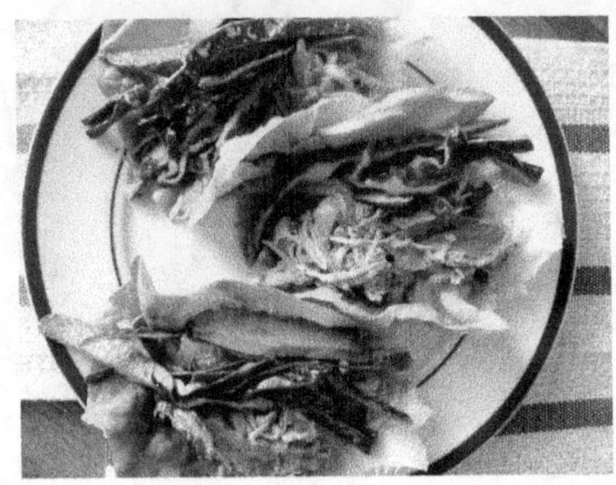

INGREDIENTS (for 6 servings)
Butter head lettuce – 1 piece
For the pork
Pork shoulder roast – 900 gr
Vegetable broth – 120 ml
Yellow onion – 1 piece
Garlic bulbets - 6 pcs
Juice of one lime
Zest and juice of one orange
Oregano – 25 gr
Cumin – 2,5 gr
Salt, pepper
For the slaw
Purple cabbage – 1 head
Dill pickles – 5-6 pcs
Yellow mustard – 5-6 tbsp
Olive oil – 30 ml
White wine vinegar – 5 ml
Salt, pepper

INSTRUCTIONS
1. Combine in a large deep saucepan all ingredients for pork. Cook it on a slow fire for 6-8 hours.
2. Take a large bowl and combine ingredients for slaw: shred the purple cabbage, slice lengthwise dill pickles, add olive oil, white wine vinegar, salt, pepper and mustard.
3. When pork is cooked, shred it or cut into pieces.

4. Take butter lettuce leaf put shredded pork and ready slaw on it and roll up.
5. Enjoy Cuban Pork Lettuce Wraps!
Nutritional values (per serving). Carbs - 14 g, protein – 29 g, fat – 30 g, energy – 436 kcal

12. Sweet & Sour Stir Fry (Lunch)

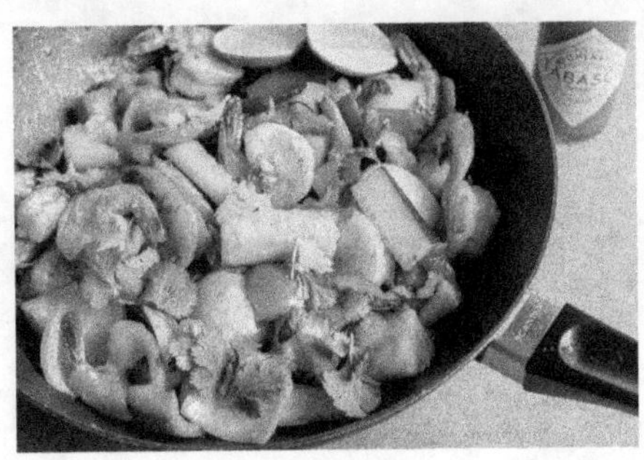

INGREDIENTS (for 3 servings)
Chicken breasts – 450 gr
Broccoli – 2 cups
Bell pepper – 1 piece
Diced pineapple – 1 can (420 gr)
Raw cashews – 40 gr
Tapioca starch – 25 gr
Green onion – 2 pcs
Coconut oil – 7 ml
For sweet and sour sauce
Pineapple juice – 60 ml
 Coconut aminos – 50 ml
Rice wine vinegar – 30 ml
Tomato paste – 50 gr
Fresh ginger – 25 gr

INSTRUCTIONS
1. Make preparations: cut chicken breasts and broccoli into bite sized pieces, deseed bell pepper and cut into chunks, dice green onion and dissolve tapioca starch in 1 tablespoon of water. Make sauce: combine all sauce ingredients. Mix well. Sweet and sour sauce is cooked.
2. Take a large pan, heat it and melt coconut oil.
3. Put chicken pieces and fry until golden brown.
4. Add broccoli pieces, pepper, drained diced pineapple, raw cashews and sauce. Toss thoroughly.
5. Cover the pan and bring to a boil. Cook for 5 minutes.
6. After pour in dissolved tapioca starch. Let it thicken the sauce.
7. That's all! Sprinkle with diced green onions!
Nutritional values (per serving)

Carbs - 46 g, protein – 51 g, fat – 25 g, energy – 609 kcal

13. Paleo Beef Enchiladas (Dinner)

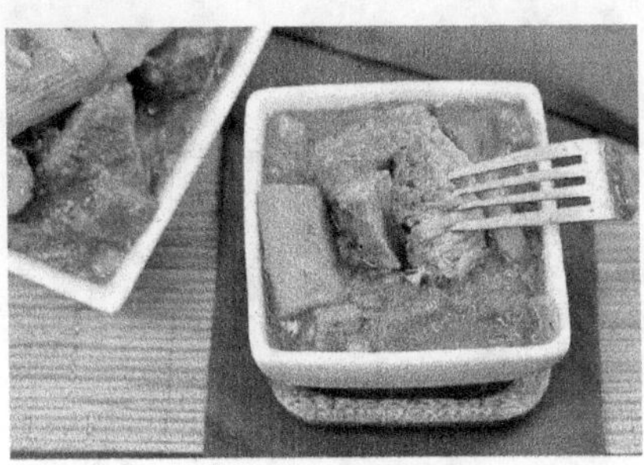

INGREDIENTS (for 4 servings)
Ground beef – 450 gr
Chicken broth – 480 ml
Paleo tortillas – 9 pcs
Extra virgin olive oil – 30 ml
Half of one onion
Jalapeno – 1 piece
Avocado – 1 piece
Fresh cilantro – 75 gr
Small onion – 1 piece
Garlic bulbets – 4 pcs
Tomato sauce – 2 cups
Chili powder – 50 gr
Cumin – 2,5 gr
Dried oregano – 1 gr
Salt
INSTRUCTIONS

1. Firstly, make enchilada sauce. Take a saucepan and heat 15 ml of olive oil. Put one half of finely diced onion and minced garlic. Sauté until soft. Add the remaining ingredients except salt . Bring to a boil and then simmer for 15-20 minutes, until sauce is thickened. Salt to taste. Make puree. Sauce is ready.
2. Second, take a pan and heat 15 ml of oil. Add the rest diced onion and fry for 4-5 minutes.
3. Add ground beef and minced jalapeno to fried onion. Salt and pepper to taste. Fry until ground beef is browned. Turn off the oven and set aside the pan. Stir in enchilada sauce.
4. Preheat the oven to176 C. Take a baking dish and spread enchilada sauce on the bottom.
5. Take tortillas and put meat mixture on each, then roll over.
6. Place rolled tortillas in the greased baking dish. Pour the remaining sauce on the top and bake for 15 minutes.
7. Serve hot! Top with chopped avocado and cilantro.
Nutritional values (per serving)

Carbs - 71 g, protein – 48 g, fat – 32 g, energy – 762 kcal

14. Paleo Sushi with Salmon & Avocado

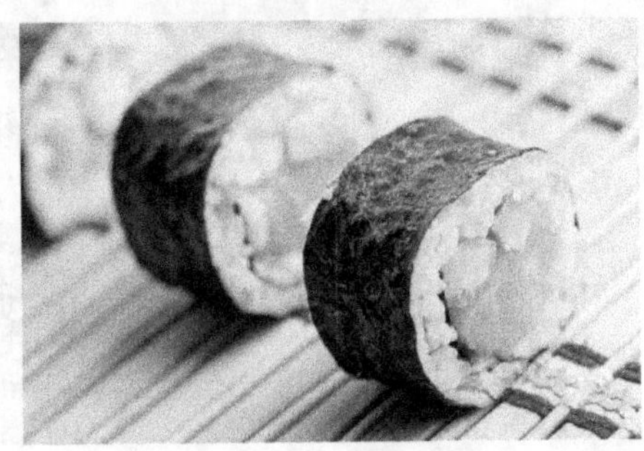

INGREDIENTS (for 4 servings)
Salmon fillet – 1 piece
Half of one red onion
Long continental cucumbers – 2 pcs
Avocado – 1 piece
Coconut aminos and wasabi
Sea salt and pepper
Coconut oil

INSTRUCTIONS
1.Spice salmon fillets with sea salt and pepper. Heat some oil in a frying pan and fry fillets brown (1-2 minutes) on both sides. Then turn fried fillets onto the dish. Let cool and mix with finely diced red onion.
2. Cut cucumbers into two cm thick rolls. Carefully cut out the flesh of the cucumber. Then fill each cucumber roll with cooked salmon-onion mixture. Top with roughly chopped avocado.
3. Put rolls in the fridge. Serve with coconut aminos and wasabi.
Nutritional values (per serving)
Carbs - 10 g, protein – 10 g, fat – 18 g, energy – 233 kcal

15. Paleo Chicken Fingers (Dinner)

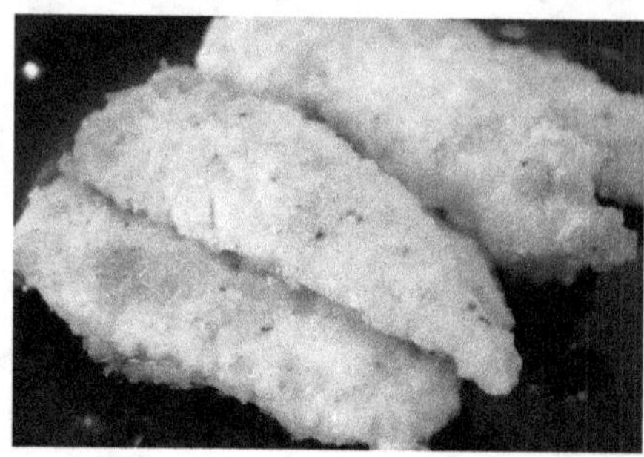

INGREDIENTS (for 6 servings)
Chicken tenderloins – 900 gr
Almond flour – 125 gr
Tapioca starch – 75 gr
Italian seasoning – 10 gr
Egg – 2 pcs
Coconut oil – 80 gr
Paprika – 2,5 gr
Black pepper – 1 gr
Garlic salt
Salt – 5 gr

INSTRUCTIONS
1. Prepare chicken. Combine dry ingredients in a bowl. Whisk eggs.
2. Heat the pan, pour 60 ml of oil. Dip each tenderloin into the egg mixture and then coat each with dry almond mixture.
3. Place chicken tenderloin into the hot pan and fry brown on both sides. During frying, dust chicken with paprika.
4. Serve with your favorite sauce or with spaghetti squash.
Nutritional values (per serving)
Carbs - 6 g, protein – 34 g, fat – 10 g, energy – 243 kcal

16. Simple Grilled Fruit Skewers Recipe (Breakfast)

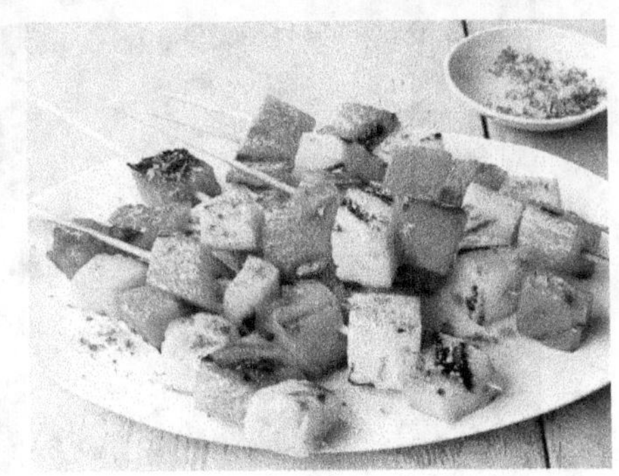

INGREDIENTS (for 4 servings)
Peach – 4 pcs
Strawberry – 1 cup
Fresh pineapple – 2 cups
Wood skewers (soaked for an hour in water)
Olive oil
Sea salt
Melted dark chocolate

INSTRUCTIONS
1. Slice peaches and cut into cubes fresh pineapple.
2. Heat your grill.
3. Thread peaches slices, strawberries, pineapple cubes on the skewers.
4. Drizzle with olive oil and if desired, season with salt.
5. Grill fruits during 8 minutes. Don't forget to flip skewers every two minutes.
6. Cover with melted dark chocolate.
Nutritional values (per serving)
Carbs – 31 g, protein – 2 g, fat – 3 g

17. Paleo Shrimp Scampi

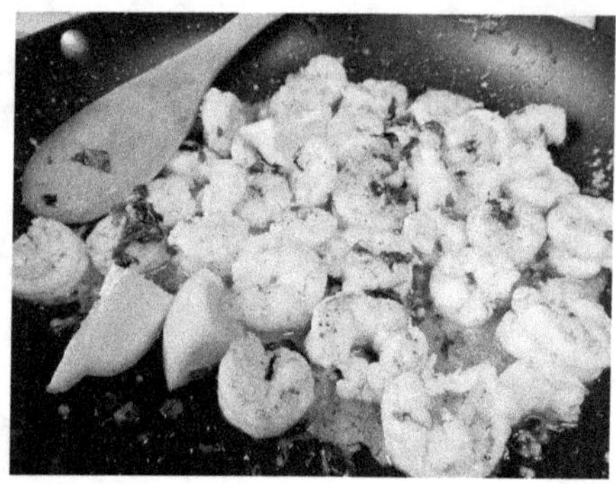

INGREDIENTS (for 6 servings)
Arrowroot flour – 32 gr
Sea salt – 2,5 gr
Ground black pepper
Paprika – 1 gr
Cayenne pepper – 1 gr
Bacon fat – ½ cup
Fresh shrimp – 900 gr
Garlic bulbets – 5 pcs
Shallot – 1 piece
Fresh parsley – ½ cup
Dried oregano – 2,5 gr
Chicken broth – 80 ml
Fresh lemon juice – 80 ml
Lemon zest – 2 gr
Sea salt, black pepper
Lemon wedges (optional)

INSTRUCTIONS
1. Wash shrimps and dry with paper towel. Lay aside.
2. Combine dry ingredients and mix well. Dip each peeled shrimp in this spicy mixture. Set shrimps aside.
3. Take a large pan and melt bacon fat. Put shrimps and fry on both sides for 4 minutes. Turn fried shrimps on the dish.
4. Put minced garlic, dried oregano and chopped fresh parsley to the pan. Cover and cook for two minutes.

5. Open and pour chicken broth and fresh lemon juice. Bring to the boiling point. Cook for one minute and then put the lemon zest. Mix carefully. Put sea salt, ground black pepper to taste.
6. Remove the pan and dip shrimps. Take out shrimps and place on the plate.
7. Top with chopped fresh parsley and lemon wedges (optional).
Nutritional values (per serving)
Carbs - 4 g, protein – 35 g, fat – 20 g, energy – 350 kcal

18. Korean-Style Short Ribs

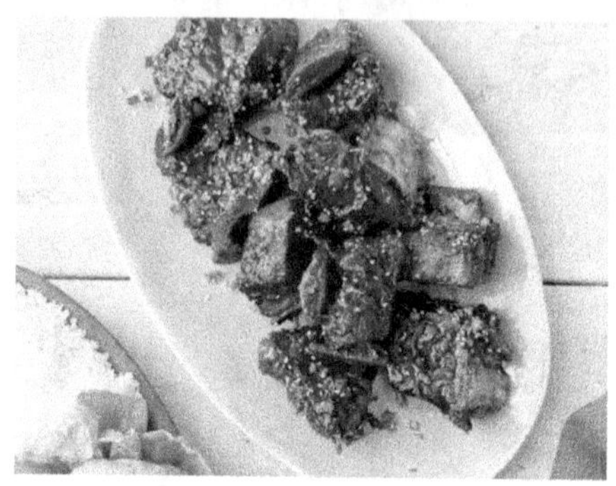

INGREDIENTS (for 4 servings)
Coconut aminos – ½ cup
Coconut sugar – ½ cup
Sesame oil – 30 ml
Rice vinegar- 30 ml
Fresh ginger – 25 gr
Garlic bulbets – 4 pcs
Crushed red pepper flakes – 0,5 tsp
Beef short ribs - 1,450 kg
For glaze:
Tapioca starch – 45 gr
Shredded carrots – 1,5 cup
Green onion – 3 pcs
Sesame seeds 25 gr

INSTRUCTIONS
1. Take a owl and combine ½ cup of coconut aminos, ½ cup of coconut sugar, 30 ml of sesame oil, 30 ml of rice vinegar, 25 gr of fresh ginger, minced garlic and 0,5 tsp of crushed red pepper. Your sauce is ready.
2. Place beef short ribs in the bottom of your saucepan and pour ready sauce on the top.
3. Cove the saucepan r and cook 4-6 hours.
4. Remove beef short ribs from the saucepan and lay aside.
5. Combine 45 gr of tapioca starch and some water, and pour into the saucepan.
6. Bring to a boil, and prepare for two minutes, until thickened.
7. Then add shredded carrots, crushed green onion and pour over the ribs.
8. Top these ribs with 25 gr of sesame seeds.

7. Top with chopped fresh parsley and lemon wedges (optional).
Nutritional values (per serving)
Carbs -35, 4 g, protein – 42 g, fat – 12 g, energy – 350 kcal

19. PEPPER STEAK

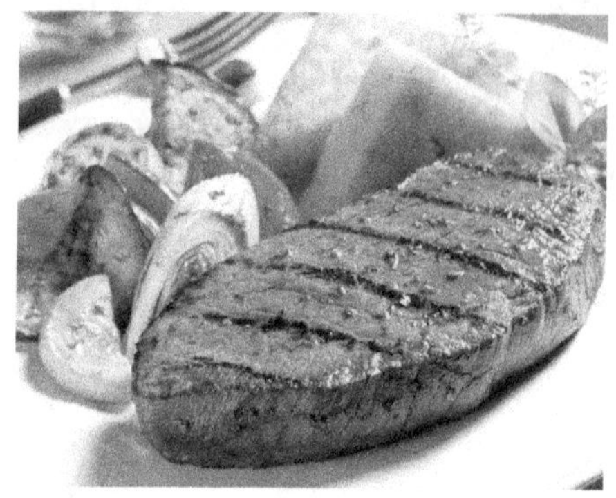

INGREDIENTS (for 4 servings)
Top round beef – 340 gr
Liquid aminos – 20 ml+55 ml
Rice wine – 15 ml
Arrowroot starch - 15 gr
Vegetable oil – 15 ml
Onion – 1 piece
Bell pepper – 1 piece
Black pepper – 5 gr
Crushed red pepper flakes

INSTRUCTIONS
1. Take beef and cut into thin slices. Combine in a bowl 20 ml of liquid aminos, 15 ml of rice wine, 1o gr of arrowroot starch and 5 gr of black pepper. Mix thoroughly and put there beef slices. Let marinate.
2. In a separate bowl, combine 55ml of liquid aminos, 18ml of water and 10 gr arrowroot starch. Set aside.
3. Take a wok, heat it and pour oil. Transfer marinated beef slices into the wok and cook until golden brown (don't forget to stir meat) letting the beef brown. After 2 minutes transfer fried beef to a plate.
4. Add oil to wok again, and spread sliced into thin strips bell pepper and onion. Fry 4- 5 minutes. Add beef, sauce and crushed red pepper flakes to the wok. Let fry 30 seconds.
5. Remove from the heat and enjoy!
Nutritional values (per serving - serving size - 1/4th of recipe)
Carbs - 12 g, protein – 22 g, fat – 6 g, energy – 187 kcal

20. CHICKEN AND SHRIMP LAAP

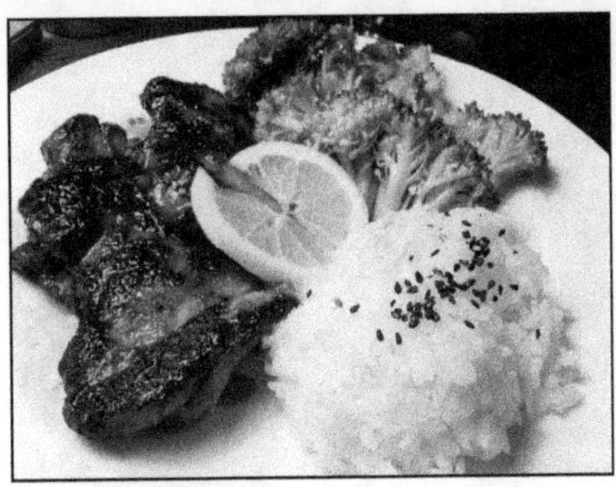

INGREDIENTS (for 4 servings)
Coconut flour – 10 gr
Oil – 5 gr
Shallot – 1 piece
Ground chicken thighs – 450 gr
Large shrimp – 225 gr
Asian fish sauce – 50-60 gr
Fresh lime juice – 30 ml
Cayenne pepper – 5 gr
Scallions – 2 pcs
Chopped cilantro – ¼ cup
Fresh mint leaves – ¼ cup
Butter lettuce – 1 head

INSTRUCTIONS
1. Preheat the oven to 150 C. Line baking tray with parchment and dust the coconut flour. Toast flour until golden brown. (You can also fry the coconut flour in a dry pan). Remove and set aside.
2. Next fry sliced shallot until softened.
3. Add the ground chicken to the shallots. Cook for 3 to 5 minutes.
4. While chicken is frying, peel shrimps and chop coarsely. Add shrimps to ground chicken and cook 2 - 3 minutes.
5. Transfer cooked chicken and shrimps into the dish, add Asian fish sauce, fresh lime juice, toasted coconut flour, and cayenne pepper. Mix.
6. Sprinkle laap with chopped cilantro and fresh mint leaves.
7. Take a lettuce leaf, put 1/3 cup of laap in it and wrap. Enjoy this spicy chicken and shrimp laap.
Nutritional values (per serving - serving size -3 rolls)

Carbs - 5 g, protein – 34 g, fat – 6,5 g, energy – 220 kcal

21. Tangy Asparagus Chicken Skillet with Roasted Carrots

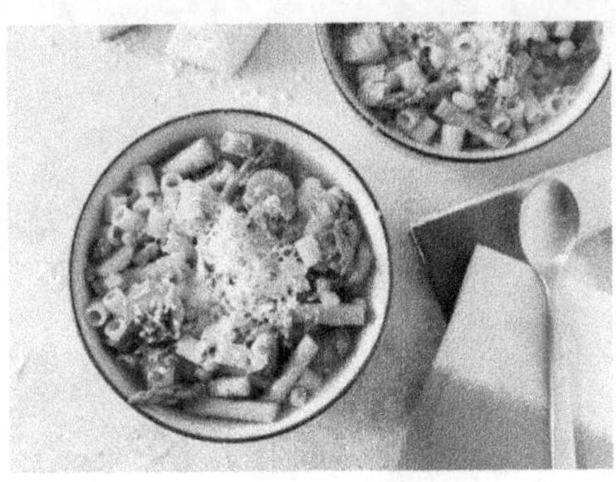

INGREDIENTS (for 2 servings)
Chicken breast – 350 gr
Carrot – 1 piece
Chopped asparagus – 1 cup
White vinegar – 5 g
Olive oil – 15 ml
Dried rosemary – 10 gr
Garlic powder – 5 gr
Lemon juice – 2 ml
Lemon zest – 5 gr
Almond flour – 25 gr
Homemade chicken stock – 120 ml
Minced garlic – 10 gr
Salt, ground black pepper

INSTRUCTION
1. Remove skin from chicken breast and cut into cubes. Put into the bowl and add there almond flour, salt, pepper to taste, lemon zest, garlic powder according to the recipe. Mix.
2. Heat the pan and 2 teaspoons of oil. Transfer chicken pieces in the pan and fry for 3 minutes. Turn out the chicken and set aside.
3. Put minced garlic and chopped asparagus into the pan and toast for 3 minutes. Pour in the homemade chicken stock, white vinegar and stir. Transfer chicken cubes back into the pan and simmer for 15 minutes.
4. While chicken is simmering, take a separate bowl and combine 5ml of olive oil, dried rosemary and julienned carrots. Toss these ingredients together. Spread carrots in the lined pan and bake in the oven for 15 minutes. When the carrots are soft, turn them out of the oven. Chill for 10 minutes.
5. Squeeze fresh lemon juice on the cooked chicken cubes and stir. Remove chicken from the pan and put on the serving plate. Spread carrots around and enjoy immediately!

Nutritional values (per serving)
Carbs - 20 g, protein – 40 g, fat – 6 g, energy – 260 kcal

22. GRILLED SALMON WITH AVOCADO BRUSCHETTA

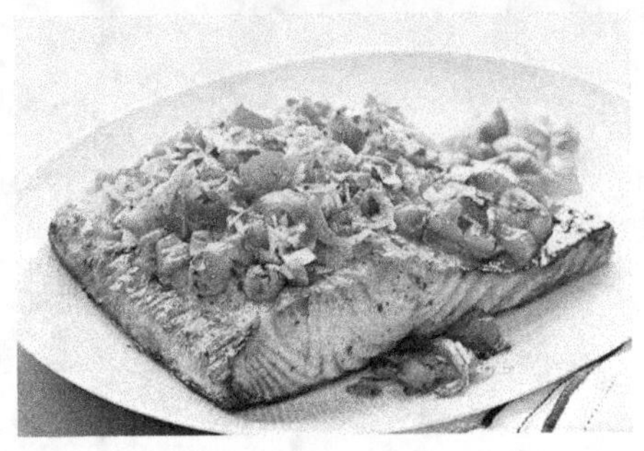

INGREDIENTS (for 4 servings)
Wild salmon filets – 4 pcs (1x140 gr)
Kosher salt
Black pepper
Cooking spray
<u>For the avocado bruschetta:</u>
Avocado – 115 gr
Red onion – ¼ cup (chopped)
Extra virgin oil – 15 ml
Balsamic vinegar – 15 ml
Ripe tomatoes – 2-4 pcs
Garlic bulbets – 2 pcs
Fresh basil leaves – 25 gr
Kosher salt, fresh cracked pepper

INSTRUCTION
1. In a separate bowl combine chopped red onion, olive oil, balsamic vinegar, a dash of kosher salt and pepper. Set aside.
2. Take another bowl and put there chopped ripe tomatoes, minced garlic, chopped basil leaves, onion-balsamic mixture. Add a dash of salt and pepper to taste. Set aside, let marinate for 10 minutes.
3. Take wild salmon fillets, flavor with salt and pepper. Let marinate for 5 minutes.
4. Preheat a gas grill, grease it and place marinated salmon fillets on the grill. Close it and cook for 8-10 minutes.
5. Turn grilled fillets onto a dish and cover with foil and rest for 2 to 3 minutes
6. Serve each fillet topped with a half cup of avocado bruschetta.
Nutritional values (per serving – 1 salmon fillet)
Carbs - 7 g, protein – 35,5 g, fat – 19 g, energy – 340,5 kcal

23. GRILLED SALMON KEBABS

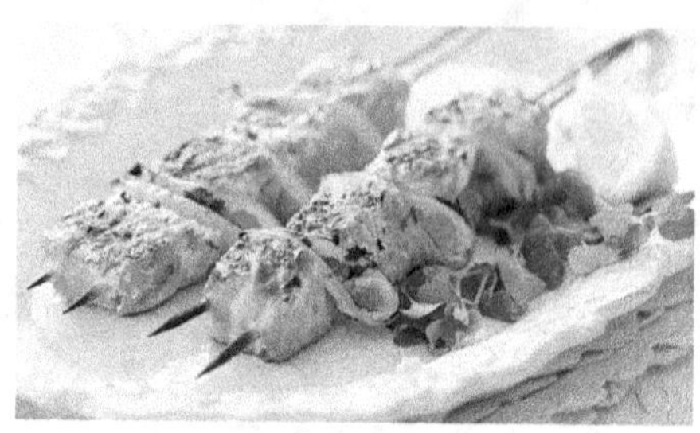

INGREDIENTS (for 4 servings)
Fresh oregano – 25 gr (chopped)
Sesame seeds – 20 gr
Ground cumin – 10 gr
Crushed red pepper flakes – 2 gr
Wild salmon fillet – 1x225 gr
Lemon – 2pcs
Olive oil
Kosher salt – 5-7 gr
Bamboo skewers – 16pcs

INSTRUCTION
1. Soak bamboo skewers in water beforehand (minimum 1 hour). Cut salmon fillets into 1-inch pieces, slice lemons into thin rounds.
2. Heat the grill and grease with olive oil.
3. In a separate bowl combine chopped fresh oregano, sesame seeds, ground cumin, and crushed red pepper flakes. Set aside.
4. Thread salmon pieces and lemon rounds onto 8 pairs of parallel bamboo skewers (NOTE begin and end with salmon). Make 8 kebabs.
5. Drizzle fish with oil and flavor with kosher salt and spice mixture.
6. Grill salmon about 8 to 10 minutes. Turn occasionally.
Nutritional values (per serving – 2 kebabs)
Carbs - 7 g, protein – 35 g, fat – 11 g, energy – 267 kcal

24. Dairy-Free Breakfast Waffles

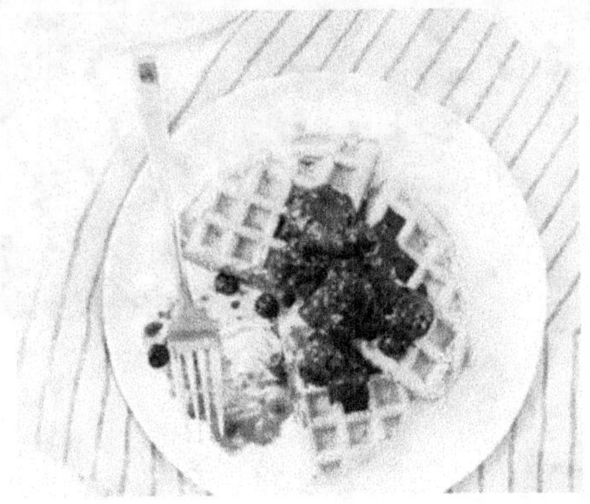

INGREDIENTS (for 4 servings)
Almond flour – 140 gr
Coconut flour – 50-60 gr
Coconut sugar – 20 gr
Eggs – 2 pcs
Baking powder – 20 gr
Apple cider vinegar – 2 ml
Olive oil – 15 ml
Almond milk – 105 ml

INSTRUCTION
1. Preheat the waffle maker and add a little cooking spray on the waffle tins.
2. Mix almond flour, coconut flour, coconut sugar and baking powder in a bowl. Set aside.
3. In a separate bowl, whisk two eggs together with the olive oil, almond milk and apple cider vinegar. Combine this mixture with dry ingredients and mix well.
4. Pour waffle batter into the waffle maker and close it. Let the waffles cook for 4 minutes or until golden brown. Transfer the waffles to a plate and serve immediately.
Nutritional values (per serving)
Carbs - 6 g, protein – 20 g, fat – 25 g, energy – 250 kcal

25. CALIFORNIA SPICY CRAB STUFFED AVOCADO

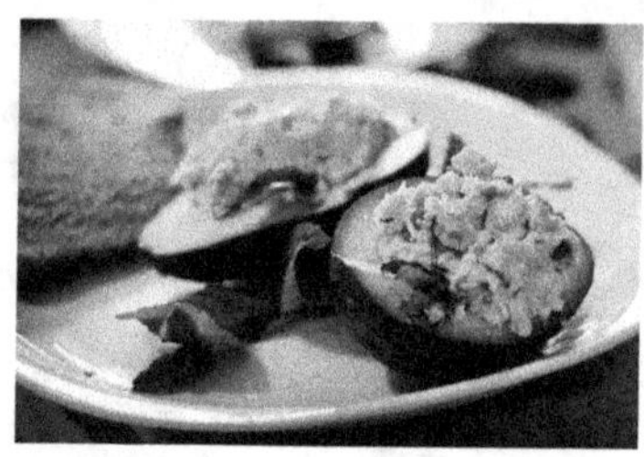

INGREDIENTS (for 2 servings)
Light mayonnaise – 50 gr
Sriracha – 20 gr
Chopped fresh chives – 10 gr
Crab meat – 115 gr
Cucumber – ¼ cup
Hass avocado – 1x115 gr (pitted and peeled)
Furikake – 5 gr
Coconut aminos – 10 gr

INSTRUCTION
1. Make preparations: chop fresh chives, peel and dice cucumber, cut avocado in half, peel the skin remove pit and scoop out the pulp, cut crab meat.
2. Take a bowl and mix light mayonnaise, sriracha and chopped chives. Add crab meat and diced cucumber. Toss carefully.
4. Stuff the avocado halves with spicy crab salad. Dust with furikake and pour with coconut aminos.
5. Bon appetit!
 Nutritional values (per 1/2 stuffed avocado)
Carbs - 7 g, protein – 12 g, fat – 13 g, energy – 194 kcal

26. Grilled Steak With Tomatoes, Red Onion and Balsamic

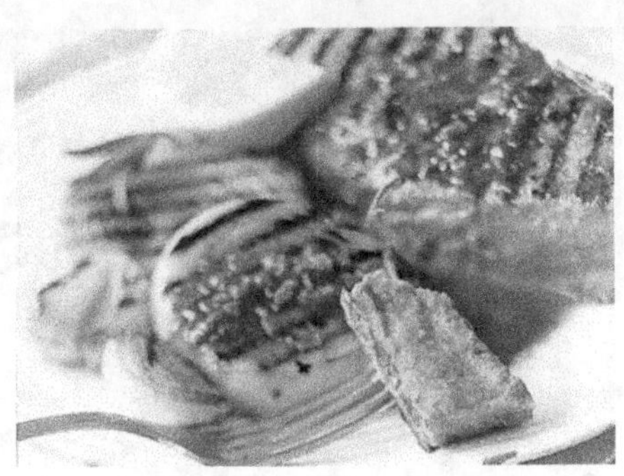

INGREDIENTS (for 8 servings)
Broil steak – 900 gr
Extra virgin olive oil – 15 ml
Balsamic – 30 ml
Red onion – 1/3 cup
Tomatoes – 3-4 pcs
Fresh herbs – 25 gr (oregano, basil, parsley)
Garlic powder
Kosher salt, fresh pepper

INSTRUCTION
1. Pierce broil steak all over with a toothpick or fork. Flavor generously with kosher salt, fresh pepper and dust with garlic powder. Marinate 10 minutes.
2. Take a large bowl, combine chopped red onion, extra virgin olive oil, balsamic, salt and pepper. Let onion to mellow a bit. Then add chopped tomatoes and fresh herbs. Taste it. Add salt and pepper if necessary.
3. Heat grill. Cook broil steak on a medium fire 7 minutes on both sides. Move steak from grill and put on the dish. Slice five minutes later.
4. Put tomatoes on the top and serve.
Nutritional values (per 85 gr steak+1/2 cup salad)
Carbs - 3 g, protein – 25 g, fat – 9 g, energy – 198 kcal

27. GRILLED PROSCIUTTO WRAPPED ASPARAGUS

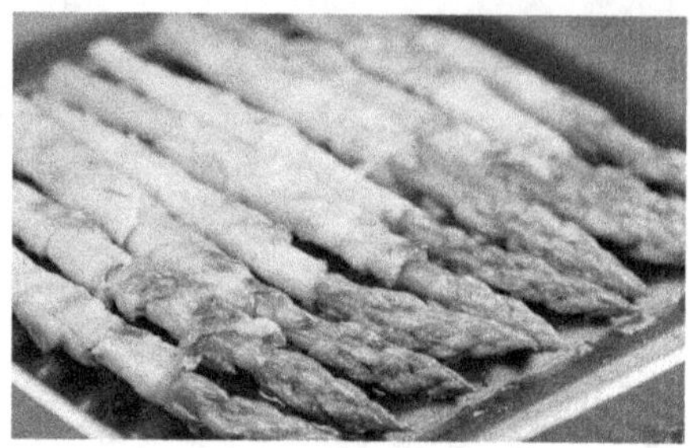

INGREDIENTS (for 4 servings)
Asparagus spears – 16 pcs (225 gr)
Prosciutto – 4 slices (56 gr)
Olive oil spray
Kosher salt
Black pepper

INSTRUCTION
1. Take asparagus spears, wash them and snap off ends. Cut each prosciutto slice into four pieces (all in all 16 pieces).
2. Wrap each prosciutto piece around the center of each asparagus spear.
3. Spray with olive oil, and season with salt and black pepper.
4. Heat grill lightly and grease with olive oil. Cook asparagus spears 5-6 minutes constantly turning.
Nutritional values (per 4 spears)
Carbs – 3,5 g, protein – 4 g, fat – 2,5 g, energy – 50 kcal

28. Garlic Shrimp in Coconut Milk, Tomatoes and Cilantro

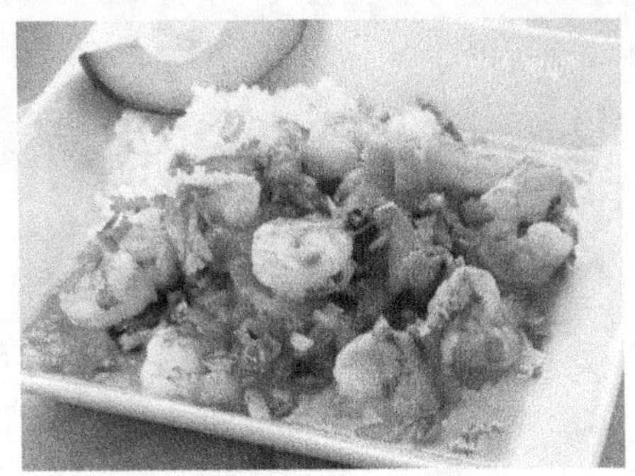

INGREDIENTS (for 4 servings)
Jumbo shrimp – 570 gr
Olive oil – 5 ml
Red bell pepper – 1 piece
Scallions – 4 pcs
Chopped cilantro – ½ cup
Garlic bulbets – 4 pcs
Crushed red pepper flakes – 4-5 gr
Diced tomatoes – 1 canx420 gr
Light coconut milk – 1 canx400 gr
Half of one lime
Kosher salt – 2 gr

INSTRUCTION
1. Make preparations: peel and devein shrimps. Dice red bell pepper, mince garlic, slice scallions and separate white and green parts.
2. Take a pot, pour oil and heat it. Add diced red peppers and fry until soft (4 minutes).
3. Add white parts of sliced scallion, ¼ cup of chopped cilantro, minced garlic and crushed red pepper flakes. Cook all together 1 minute. Then add diced tomatoes, pour in coconut milk and a dash of salt. Bring this mixture to a boil, cover and simmer for 10 minutes until thicken. Sauce is ready.
4. Add shrimps and cook only 5-6 minutes. Squeeze lime.
5. Divide into four equal parts (about 1 ¼ cups)
6. Serve topped with green parts of scallions and chopped cilantro.
Nutritional values (per 1 ½ cups)
Carbs – 9,5 g, protein – 30 g, fat – 10,5 g, energy – 267 kcal

29. Chicken and Mushrooms in a Garlic White Wine Sauce

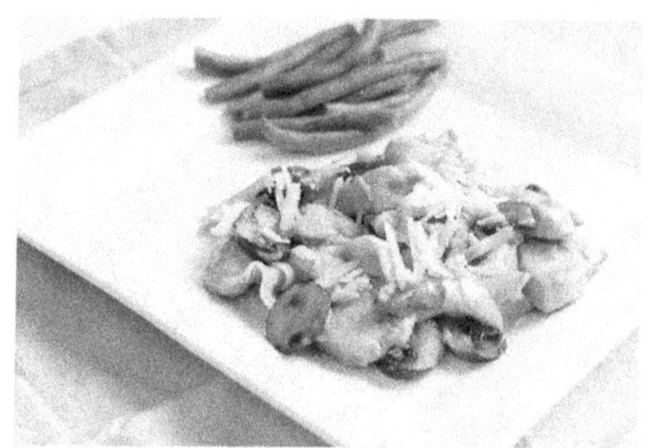

INGREDIENTS (for 8 tenderloins)
Chicken tenderloins – 8 pcs (450 gr)
Butter – 20 gr
Olive oil – 10 ml
Garlic bulbets – 3 pcs
Mushrooms – 340 gr
Defatted chicken broth – 120 ml
Chopped fresh parsley – 35 gr
Salt and fresh pepper

INSTRUCTION
1. Firstly preheat oven to 95 C. Salt and pepper chicken tenderloins.
2. Heat a large pan, add 10 gr of butter and 5 ml of oil. Put chicken and fry for 5 minutes per side.
3. Add oil and butter to the pan and fry minced garlic for 10-15 seconds; put sliced mushrooms, salt and pepper and cook for 5 minutes.
4. Pour in defatted chicken broth, chopped fresh parsley. Cook until the liquid evaporates by half.
5. Put tenderloins on the dish and pour with the mushroom sauce on the top. Enjoy!
Nutritional values (per two tenderloins with mushrooms)
Carbs – 6 g, protein – 29,5 g, fat – 7,5 g, energy – 217 kcal

30. GRILLED CHICKEN BRUSCHETTA

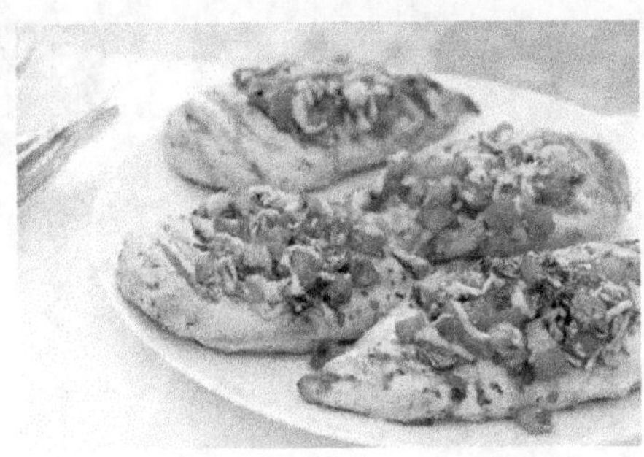

INGREDIENTS (for 4 servings)
Vine ripe tomatoes – 3 pcs
Garlic bulbets – 2 pcs
Chopped red onion – ¼ cup
Chopped fresh basil leaves – 50 gr
Extra virgin oil – 15 ml
Balsamic vinegar – 15 ml
Chicken cutlets – 700 gr (8 pcs)
Kosher salt, fresh cracked pepper

INSTRUCTION
1. In a separate bowl combine such ingredients as: chopped red onion, balsamic vinegar,olive oil, kosher salt, pepper.
2. Chop tomatoes and put in another large bowl. Add minced garlic, chopped fresh basil leaves, onion-balsamic mixture. Salt and pepper the mixture. Toss, set aside (for ten minutes).
3. Preheat the grill and grease it. Season chicken cutlets with salt and fresh pepper.
4. Grill cutlets 2 minutes per side. Put grilled chicken cutlets on the platter. Top with bruschetta and enjoy!
Nutritional values (per 2 cutlets)
Carbs – 7 g, protein – 32 g, fat – 8,5 g, energy – 237 kcal

31. THE BEST ENCHILADA SAUCE RECIPE

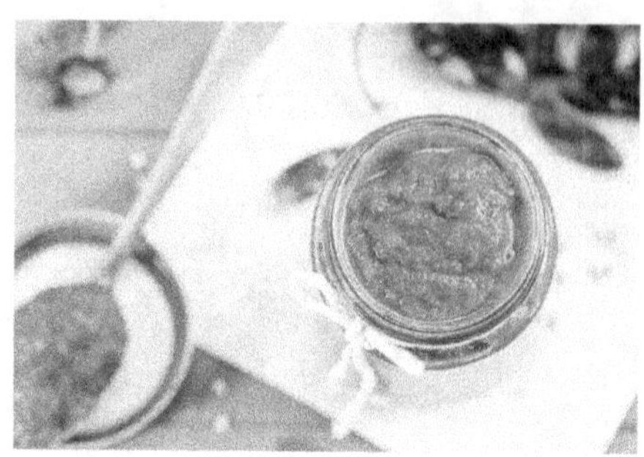

INGREDIENTS (for 16 servings)
Olive oil – 2 ml
Garlic bulbets – 4 pcs
Vegetable broth – 360 ml
Tomato sauce – 500 gr
Chopped chipotle chilis in adobo sauce – 30 gr
Mexican hot chili powder – 5gr
Ground cumin – 5 gr
Kosher salt – 2 gr
Fresh black pepper

INSTRUCTIONS
1. Fry minced garlic in a pan, then pour vegetable broth, add tomato sauce, chopped chipotle chilis in adobo sauce, ground cumin, Mexican hot chili powder, salt and pepper. Bring this spicy mixture to a boil, reduce heat and continue to simmer for 7-10 minutes.
2. The best Enchilada sauce is ready.
Nutritional values (per ¼ cup)
Carbs – 4 g, protein – 1 g, fat – 0 g, energy – 20 kcal

32. Mixed Baby Greens with Strawberries, Gorgonzola and Poppy Seed Dressing

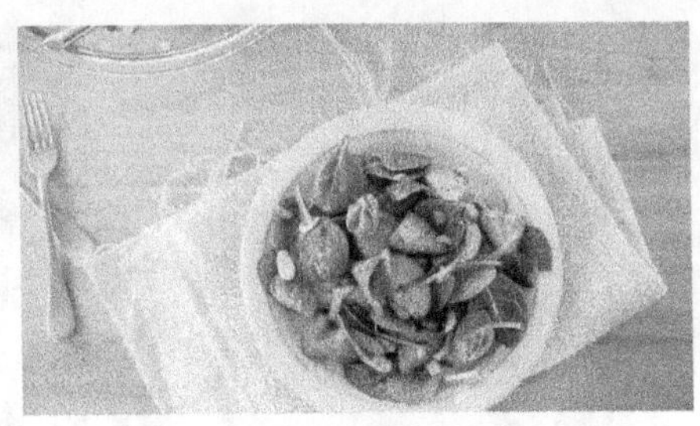

INGREDIENTS (for 4 servings)
For the dressing:
Red wine vinegar – 15ml
Cider vinegar – 15 ml
Olive oil – 30 ml
Minced shallots – 10 gr
Raw honey – 45 gr
Poppy seeds – 15gr
For the salad:
Organic mixed baby greens – 140 gr
Slivered almond – ¼ cup
Sliced strawberries – 2 cups

INSTRUCTIONS
1. Combine all ingredients for the dressing in a small clean jar. Shake well.
2. Take a platen and combine all ingredients for the salad. Mix and add dressing. Toss well.
Nutritional values (per ¼ of recipe)
Carbs – 16,5 g, protein – 5 g, fat – 14 g, energy – 198 kcal

33. SHOYU AHI POKE

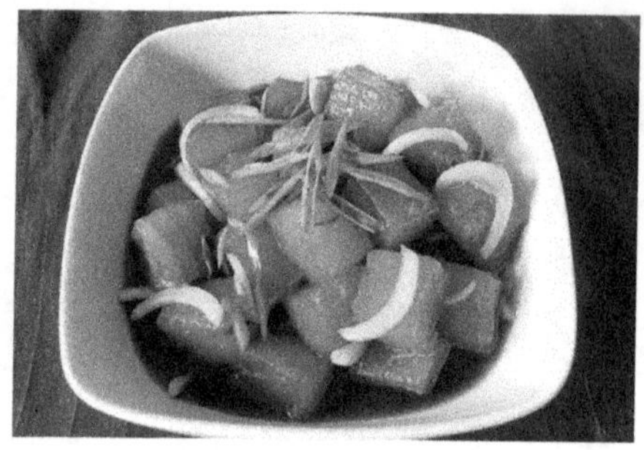

INGREDIENTS (for 4 servings)
Sushi grade tuna – 450 gr
Onion – ¼ cups
Scallions – 1/2cup (only green parts)
Coconut aminos – 30 ml
Sesame oil – 5 ml
Sriracha – 2 ml

INSTRUCTIONS
1. Cut tuna into cubes, slice onion and scallions.
2. Take a bowl and mix all ingredients together.
3. Serve immediately!
Nutritional values (per 115 gr)
Carbs – 2,5 g, protein – 28,5 g, fat – 4 g, energy – 166 kcal

34. Sheet Pan Shrimp with Broccolini and Tomatoes

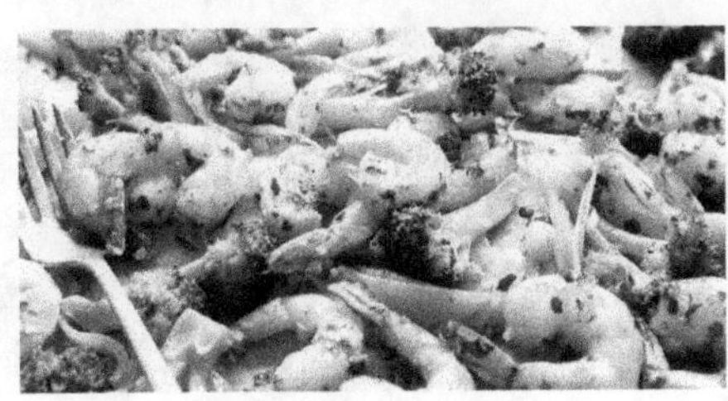

INGREDIENTS (for 4 servings)
Large shrimp – 450 gr (28 pcs)
Extra-virgin olive oil – 30 ml+10ml
Garlic bulbets – 3 pcs
Broccolini – 340 gr (12 spears)
Grape tomatoes – 1 cup
Chopped fresh oregano – 10 gr
Fresh lemon juice – 30 ml
Kosher salt
Crushed red pepper flakes
Black pepper
Olive oil

INSTRUCTIONS
1. Preheat oven to 200C. Peel and divine shrimps, pick off tails. Cut tomatoes in halve.
2. In a separate bowl combine 10 ml of olive oil, minced garlic, salt, crushed red pepper flakes and black pepper. Roll shrimps in this mixture and set aside.
3. Take a sheet pan and grease with oil. Place broccolini and tomatoes halves on the pan, add 30 ml of olive oil, a dash of salt, black pepper and chopped fresh oregano. Cook for 15 minutes (stir constantly).
4. Spread shrimps around the veggies. Cook for 8 minutes.
5. Sprinkle with fresh lemon juice. Serve.
Nutritional values (per 7 shrimps, 3 spears broccolini+tomatoes)
Carbs – 9 g, protein – 26 g, fat – 11,5 g, energy – 238 kcal

35. FILIPINO ADOBO CHICKEN

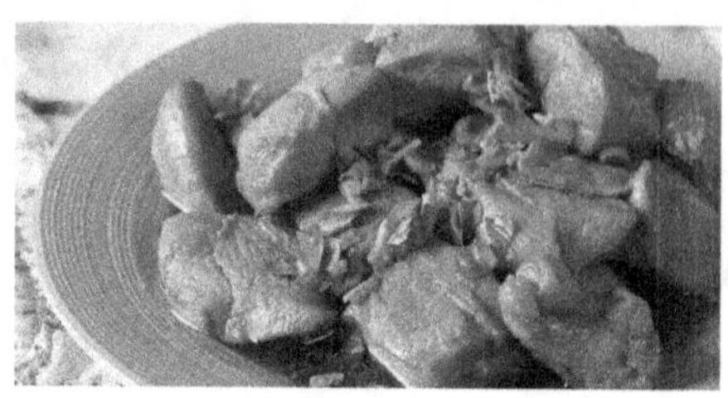

INGREDIENTS (for 4 servings)
Chicken drumsticks (on the bone) – 8 pcs
Coconut aminos – 80 ml
Apple cider vinegar – 80 ml
Water – 120 ml
Head of garlic – 1 piece
Ground peppercorns – 6 pcs
Bay leave – 4 pcs
Jalapeño – 1 piece

INSTRUCTIONS
1. To make marinade: combine apple cider vinegar, coconut aminos, crushed garlic, chopped jalapeño and ground peppercorns. Mix thoroughly.
2. Marinate skinless chicken drumsticks in marinade for overnight.
3. Take a pan and pour 120 ml of water, marinade, put bay leaves and add marinated drumsticks. Cook on the medium fire for an hour. Until chicken is tender.
4. Open the pan and cook for another 15 minutes.
5. Filipino adobo chicken is ready. Serve with rice.
Nutritional values (per 2 drumsticks)
Carbs – 5 g, protein – 27 g, fat – 4,5 g, energy – 175 kcal

36. Grilled Zesty Sweet Potatoes Recipe

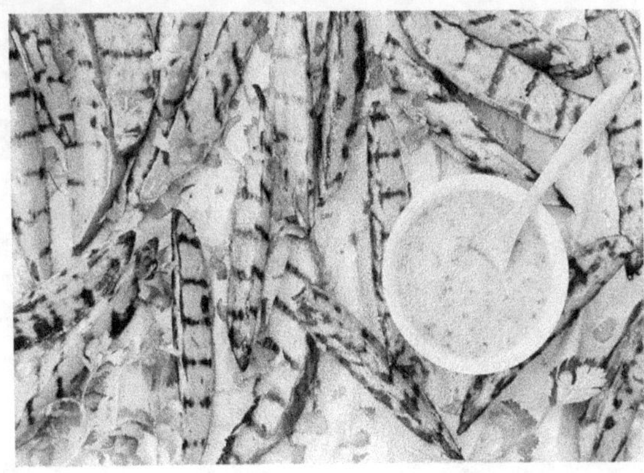

INGREDIENTS (for 4 servings)
Sweet potato – 5 pcs
Fresh parsley – ¼ cup
Lemon zest – 10 gr
Fresh lemon juice – 30 ml
Garlic bulbets – 2 pcs
Olive oil – 60 ml + 60 ml
Sea salt, ground black pepper

INSTRUCTIONS
1. Cut sweet potatoes into slices, mince parsley and garlic.
2. Heat grill in advance.
3. Mix olive oil, salt and pepper in a bowl. Put in sweet potato slices and toss well.
4. In a separate bowl make lemon dressing. Combine minced parsley, lemon zest, fresh lemon juice, minced garlic and olive oil. Whisk.
5. Grill sweet potatoes for 5 minutes on both sides.
6. Transfer grilled sweet potatoes into a bowl with lemon dressing. Mix well.
Nutritional values (per serving)
Carbs – 33 g, protein – 3 g, fat – 27 g

37. BURGER BITES

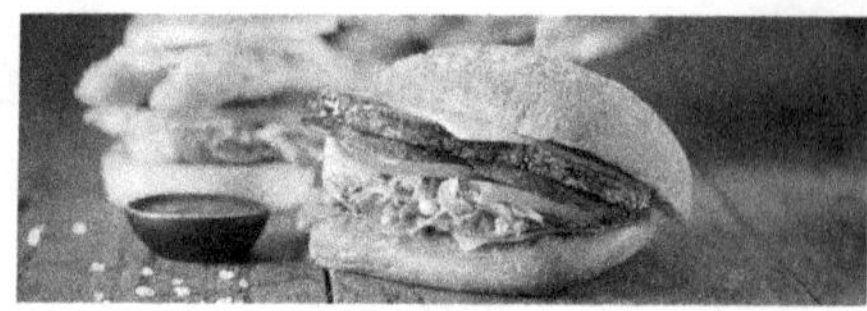

INGREDIENTS (for 30 "bites")
Beef - 900 gr
Raw bacon 45 gr
Mustard – 30 ml
Butter lettuce – 1 head
Cherry tomatoes – 30 pcs
Dill pickle chips – 30 pcs
Kosher salt – 2 gr
Onion powder – 2 gr
Black pepper – 1 gr
Ketchup, mayonnaise

INSTRUCTIONS
1. Put into a bowl beef, minced raw bacon, mustard, kosher salt, onion powder and black pepper.Mix thoroughly.
2. Make 30 small meatballs.
3. Fry each meatball on the preheated greased grill pan for 3 minutes both sides.
4. Place fried meatballs on skewers, add lettuce, dill pickle chips and cherry tomatoes. Optionally dip in ketchup, mustard or mayonnaise.
5. Bon appetite!
Nutritional values (per 1 bite)
Carbs – 1,5 g, protein – 8 g, fat – 2,5 g, energy – 66 kcal

38. Roasted Cauliflower "Rice" with Garlic and Lemon

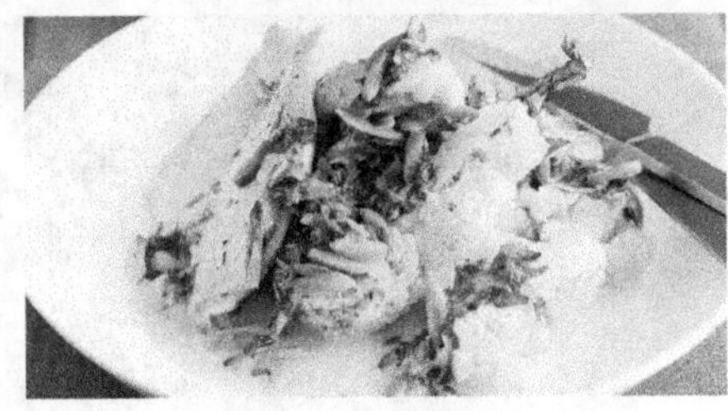

INGREDIENTS (for 2 servings)
Riced cauliflower – 450 gr
Olive oil – 15 ml
Garlic bulbets – 3
Fresh chopped parsley – 20 gr
Fresh lemon juice – 5 ml
Kosher salt – 1 gr

INSTRUCTIONS
1. Preheat oven to 220C. Grease a baking tray with oil.
2. Spread riced cauliflower, olive oil, chopped garlic on the baking tray. Dust with salt. Bake for 25 minutes until golden.
3. Take the tray out, drizzle with fresh lemon juice and fresh chopped parsley.
Nutritional values (per 3/4 cup)
Carbs – 13,5 g, protein – 5 g, fat – 7 g, energy – 124 kcal

39. SLOPPY JOE BAKED SWEET POTATOES

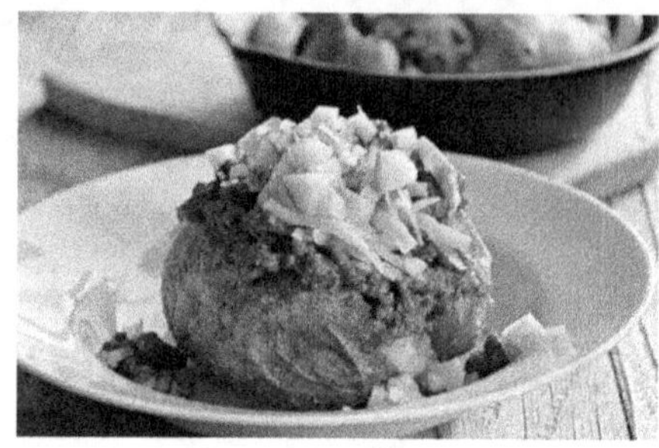

INGREDIENTS (for 4 Servings)
Sweet potato – 4 pcs (200 gr each potato)
Lean ground beef – 225 gr
Chopped carrot – 50 gr
Chopped onion – 50 gr
Chopped mushrooms – 50 gr
Chopped red bell pepper – 50 gr
Garlic bulbet – 1 piece
Red wine vinegar – 15 ml
Worcestershire sauce – 15 ml
Tomato sauce – 1 can x 225 gr
Tomato paste – 50 gr
Water – 80 ml
Chopped scallion – 1 piece
Salt – 5 gr

INSTRUCTIONS :
1. Pierce each potato with a fork. Cook in microwave oven for 7 -10 minutes.
2. Heat a pan and put ground beef. Salt to taste. Then put chopped vegetables. Mix.
3. Slack the fire, pour in 15 ml of red wine vinegar and 15 ml of Worcestershire sauce. Cook 4-5 minutes more. Add 225 gr of tomato sauce, 50 gr of tomato paste and pour in 80 ml of water to the skillet. Stir.
4. Cover and simmer at medium heat 15 -20 minutes.
5. Cut sweet potatoes and place on the dish. Add a pinch of salt and garnish each potato with 1/2 cup of meat and chopped scallion.
Nutritional values (per 200 gr potato, ½ cup meat)
Carbs – 40 g, protein – 15,5 g, fat – 4 g, energy – 259 kcal

40. Brussels Sprouts and Sausage Parsnip Spiralized Pasta

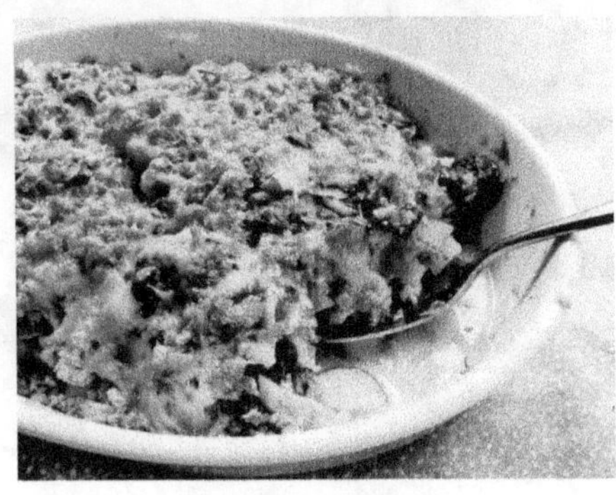

INGREDIENTS (for 2 servings)
Chicken Italian Sausage - 2 links
Brussels sprouts – 140 gr
Olive oil – 10 gr
Parsnip – 1 large
Chopped shallots – ¼ cup
Garlic bulbets – 2 pcs
Crushed red pepper flakes – ¼ tsp
Chicken broth – 120 ml
Grated parmesan cheese – 50 gr
Kosher salt
Black pepper

INSTRUCTION:
1. Make preparations: shred brussels sprouts, peel parsnip and spiralize; mince garlic bulbets.
2. Preheat the pan, pour some oil and add sausages. Cook until browned. Turn sausages onto a plate.
3. Add more oil and fry shredded brussels sprouts, chopped shallots and minced garlic. Cook until golden. Turn fried veggies onto a plate.
4. Pour chicken broth in the pan, add parsnip noodles crushed red pepper flakes and simmer until parsnip noodles are al dente.
5. Add sausages and brussels to noodles, sprinkle with grated parmesan. Stir thoroughly. Brussels sprouts and Sausage Parsnip Spiralized Pasta is done! Enjoy!
Nutritional values (per 1 3/4 cup)
Carbs – 29 g, protein – 23 g, fat – 16 g, energy – 336 kcal

41. ROASTED DELICATA SQUASH WITH TURMERIC

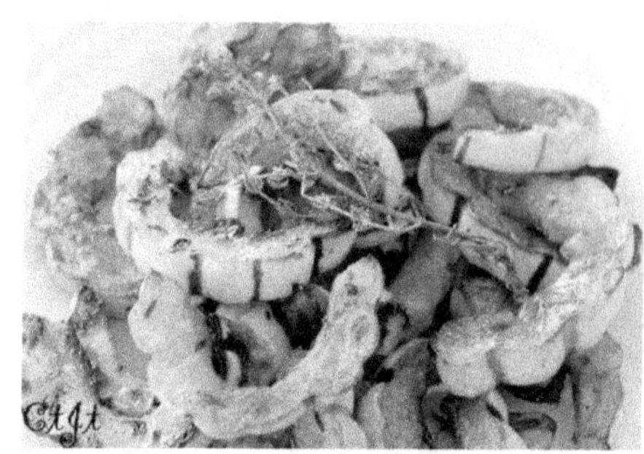

INGREDIENTS (for 4 servings)
Squash – 2 x 400gr,
Kosher salt
Ground turmeric – 3 gr
Garlic powder – 3 gr
Fresh black pepper
Chopped fresh cilantro
Cooking spray
Olive oil – 25 ml

INSTRUCTION
1. Preheat oven to 220°C. Prepare two baking sheets, spray them with oil.
2. Wash and dry squash. Cut it in half and scoop out the seeds. Slice squash into thick slices. Put in a bowl.
3. Drizzle squash slices with olive oil, kosher salt, ground turmeric, garlic powder and fresh black pepper. Toss well.
4. Lay spiced squash slices on greased baking sheets. Bake until golden brown. Don't forget to turn over them.
5. Take out roasted squash with turmeric and put on the dish. Top with fresh cilantro and eat immediately!
Nutritional values (per ½ cup)
Carbs – 21 g, protein – 2 g, fat – 5 g, energy – 126 kcal

42. GRILLED BRUSSELS SPROUTS WITH BALSAMIC GLAZE

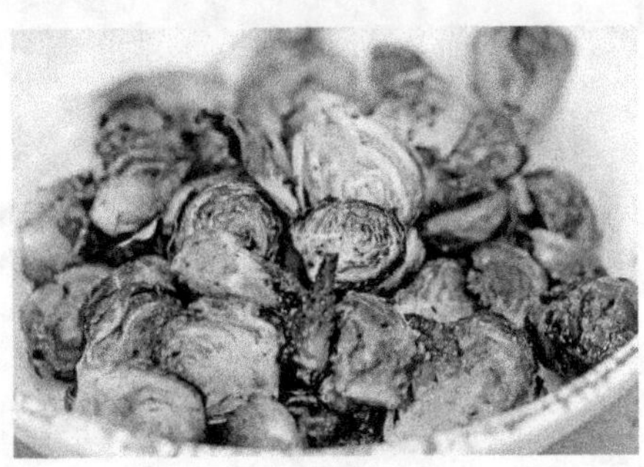

INGREDIENTS (for 4 servings)
Brussels sprouts – 450 gr
Olive oil -30 ml
Cracked black pepper
Balsamic glaze – 15 ml
Wooden skewers – 4 pcs
Kosher salt

INSTRUCTION
1. Trim stems and cut in halves brussels sprouts. Thread brussels on skewers and put them s on lined foil. Sprinkle with olive oil, add salt and pepper.
2. Heat the grill, and line foil with skewers. Cover veggies with foil. Grill for half an hour, turning every 5 minutes. Finally, sprinkle with balsamic glaze and eat immediately.
Nutritional values (per 1 skewer)
Carbs – 12,5 g, protein – 4 g, fat – 7 g, energy – 118 kcal

43. MEXICAN CAULIFLOWER "RICE"

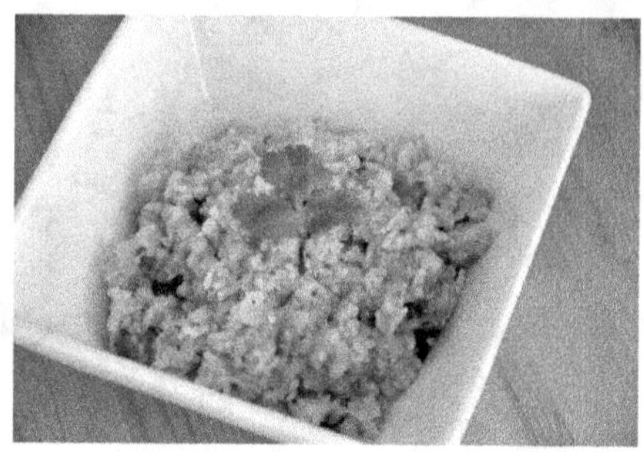

INGREDIENTS (for 4 servings)
Cauliflower crumbles – 4 cups
Onion – ½
Plum tomatoes -2 pcs
Jalapeno – 1 piece
Garlic bulbets – 2 pcs
Tomato paste – 50 gr
Cumin – 2 gr
Smoked paprika – 1 gr
Cayenne pepper – 1 gr
Kosher salt – 5 gr
Ground black pepper
Chopped cilantro
Olive oil – 5 gr

INSTRUCTIONS
1. Prepare vegetables: cut half of one onion and dice it finely, remove seeds and membranes from pepper and mince it, mince garlic and dice tomatoes into small pieces.
2. Heat the pan and add oil. Put diced onion, tomatoes, jalapeno and fry until tender. Add minced garlic and cauliflower crumbles. Fry about 2 min.
3. Two minutes late, put 50 gr of tomato paste and spices. Salt and pepper to taste. Stir well and cook 1 minute.
4. Divide into portions. Top with chopped cilantro. Serve!
Nutritional values (per 1 scant cup)
Carbs – 10 g, protein – 3 g, fat – 1,5 g, energy – 58 kcal

44. STEAK KEBABS WITH CHIMICHURRI

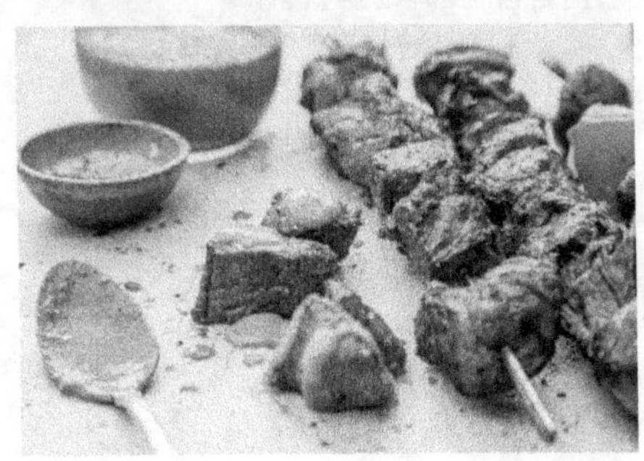

INGREDIENTS (for 6 skewers)
Beef – 600 gr
Ground pepper
Kosher salt
Red onion – 1 piece
Cherry tomatoes – 18 pcs
Bamboo skewers - 6 pcs
For chimichurri sauce:
Chopped parsley – 40 gr
Chopped cilantro – 40 gr
Chopped onion – 50 gr
Garlic bulbet – 1 piece
Extra virgin olive oil – 30 ml
Apple cider vinegar – 30 ml
Water – 15 ml
Kosher salt
 Fresh black pepper
Crushed red pepper flakes

INSTRUCTIONS
1. Salt and pepper meat. Cut into cubes.
2. Make the chimichurri sauce: combine chopped red onion, apple cider vinegar, kosher salt and olive oil. Mix and set aside for 5 minutes. Then add chopped parsley, cilantro, minced garlic, water, salt, fresh black pepper and crushed red pepper flakes. Mix together and put in the fridge for an hour.
3. Take skewers and thread onion chunks, beef cubes and tomatoes.

4. Heat the grill on high heat. Cook 2-3 minutes on both sides. Transfer steak kebabs on the plate and top with Chimichurri sauce.
Nutritional values (per 1 skewer)
Carbs – 5,5 g, protein –20 g, fat – 13 g, energy – 219 kcal

45. QUICK GARLIC LIME MARINATED PORK CHOPS

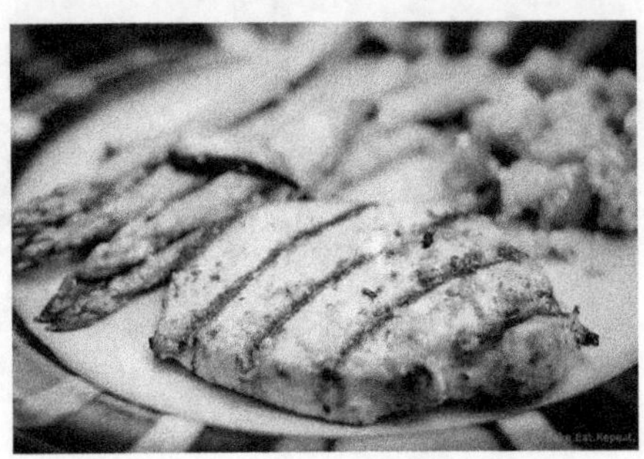

INGREDIENTS (for 4 servings)
Lean boneless pork chops – 4 pcs (170 gr each)
Garlic bulbets – 4 pcs
Cumin – 2 gr
Chili powder – 2 gr
Paprika – 2 gr
Lime juice – 10 ml
Lime zest – 2 gr
Kosher salt
Fresh pepper

INSTRUCTIONS
1. In a separate bowl combine crushed garlic, paprika, cumin, salt and pepper, chili powder. Mix well.
2. Toss pork chops in this spicy mixture. Add fresh squeezed lime juice and lime zest. Let marinate for half an hour.
3. Prepare broiler: line it with foil and place marinated pork chops. Broil 4-5 minutes per side.
4. Enjoy warm!
Nutritional values (per 1chop)
Carbs – 1,8 g, protein –38 g, fat – 6 g, energy – 224 kcal

46. Open-Faced Omelet with Avocado and Pico de Gallo

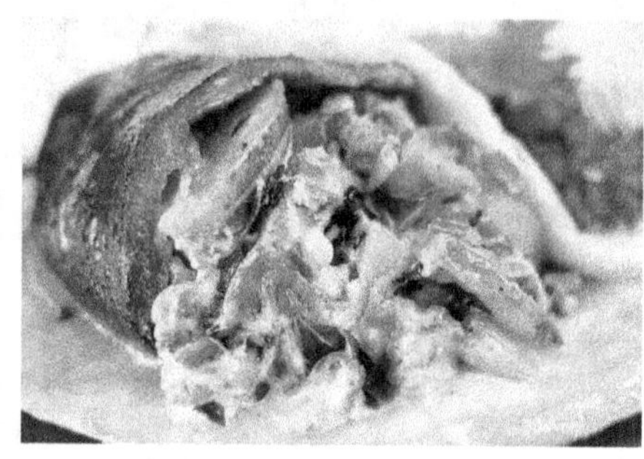

INGREDIENTS (for 1 serving)
Cooking spray
Egg– one large
Egg white – 1 large
Avocado – 1 piece (30 gr)
Pico de gallo – 30 gr
Salt, pepper

INSTRUCTIONS
1. Whisk one large egg and one egg white. Add salt and pepper to taste.
2. Heat the pan, spray with oil and pour egg mixture. Cook for 2-3 minutes.
3. Ready omelet transfer on the dish. Top with avocado slices and drizzle with pico de gallo sauce!
Nutritional values (per 1 omelet)
Carbs – 4 g, protein –11 g, fat – 9 g, energy – 140 kcal

47. ROASTED RAINBOW CARROTS WITH GINGER

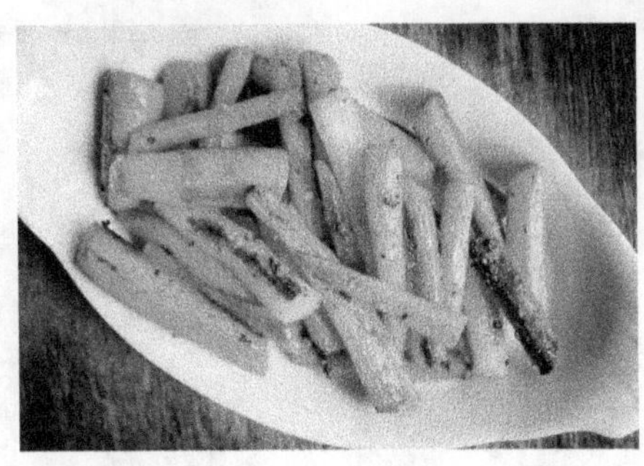

INGREDIENTS (for 6 servings)
Rainbow carrots – 1 kg
Ground black pepper
Finely minced ginger – 10 gr
Chopped cilantro – 50 gr
Olive oil – 15 ml
Kosher salt

INSTRUCTIONS
1. Heat the oven 220 C. Line the baking sheet with wax paper. Peel carrots and cut crosswise.
2. Mix together cutted carrots, olive oil, a pinch of salt, pepper and finely minced ginger.
3. Place carrots on a lined sheet and cook for half an hour. Carrots should be caramelized and soft.
 4. Drizzle roasted carrots with oil, spread cilantro. Stir and enjoy!
Nutritional values (per ½ cup)
Carbs – 15 g, protein –1 g, fat – 0,5 g, energy – 82 kcal

48. Grilled Fish Fillet in Foil Packets

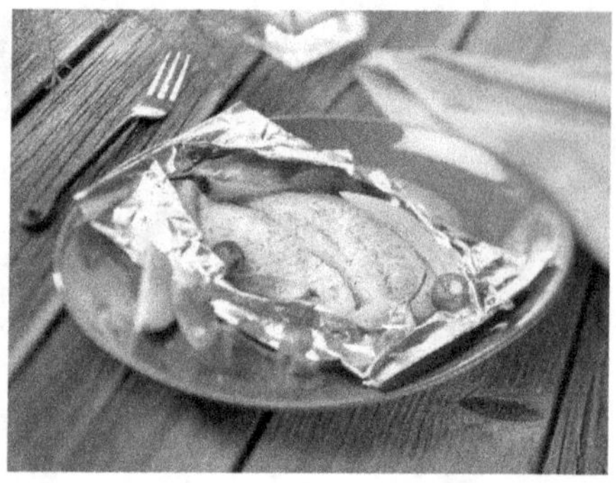

INGREDIENTS (for 4 servings)
Porgy fillets – 4 pcs (140 gr each)
Olive oil – 20 ml
Fresh herbs – 4 springs (any you like oregano, parsley, rosemary)
Lemon
Salt, fresh pepper
Foil

INSTRUCTIONS
1. Line foil and place porgy fillets in the center. Drizzle with salt, fresh pepper and olive oil. Also put lemon slices and herbs over each fillet.
2. Seal each fillet.
3. Heat the grill and place packed fish. Close it and cook 10-15 minutes.
4. Unwrap foil and enjoy juicy, flavored, tasty fish!
Nutritional values (per1 fish packet)
Carbs – 3 g, protein –27 g, fat – 8 g, energy – 194 kcal

49. BACON WRAPPED GREEN BEAN BUNDLES

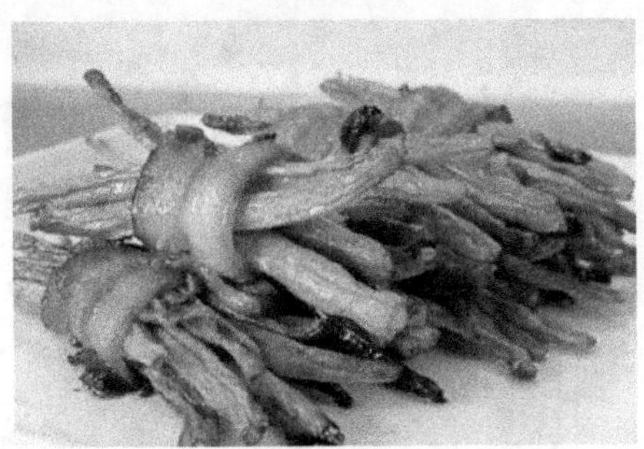

INGREDIENTS (for 4 servings)
Green beans – 450 gr (ends trimmed)
Bacon – 4 slices, cut each in half
Olive oil (spray)
Fresh cracked pepper
Salt
Garlic powder

INSTRUCTIONS
1. Dip green beans in boiling water for 3 minutes. Dry on paper towel.
2. Heat the oven to 190 C in advance. Spray your baking sheet with olive oil spray.
3. Divide beans into 8 equal bundles. Roll up each bundle in bacon slice. You will get 8 bacon wrapped bean bundles.
4. Put all bundles on the baking sheet.
5. Spray with oil again, drizzle with salt, fresh cracked pepper and dust with garlic powder.
6. Bake for about 15 min.
Nutritional values (per 2 bundles)
Carbs – 8 g, protein - 6 g, fat – 2,5 g, energy – 75,5 kcal

50. Baked Eggs with Wilted Baby Spinach

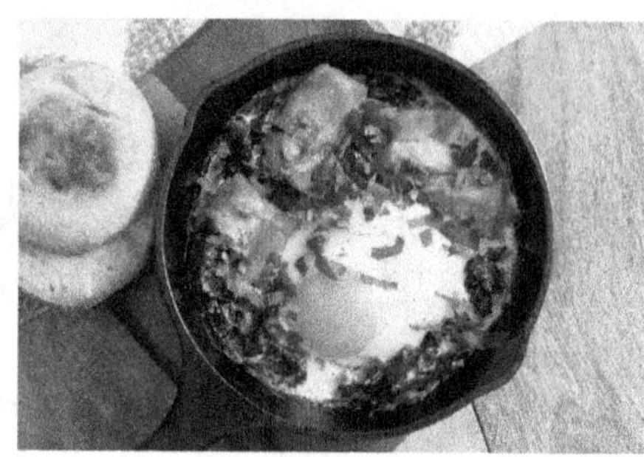

INGREDIENTS (for 4 servings)
Olive oil – 10 ml
Shallots – ¼ cup
Baby spinach – 680 gr
Egg – 4 pcs
Salt, ground pepper
Shredded Asagio cheese – 50 gr
Cooking spray

INSTRUCTIONS
1. Heat the oven to 200C. Dice shallots and shred cheese.
2. Spray four glass dishes or ramekins with oil.
3. Heat the pan and pour oil. Add diced shallots, fry 2-3 minutes. Add baby spinach, salt, ground pepper. Cook until the spinach droops. Stir in shredded Asagio cheese. Remove from the stove.
4. Divide spinach among glass dishes. Make a hole in the center of each dish and break eggs. Flavor with salt and ground pepper.
5. Bake for 17 minutes. Take out of the oven and serve immediately.
Nutritional values (per 1 egg)
Carbs – 7,9 g, protein – 12,2 g, fat – 9,3 g, energy – 152,5 kcal

51. Deviled Eggs With Bacon Recipe

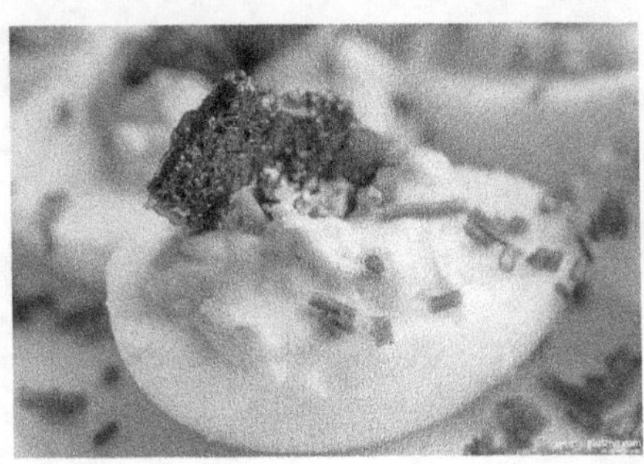

INGREDIENTS (for 4 servings)
Egg – 12 pcs
Bacon slices – 6 pcs
Mayonnaise – ½ cup
Dijon mustard – 25 gr
Paprika – 5 gr
Fresh parsley
Sea salt, ground black pepper

INSTRUCTIONS
1. Boil eggs and then peel.
2. Fry the bacon until crispy. Mince fried bacon into tiny pieces.
3. Cut eggs in half and remove all yolks.
4. Mash egg yolks with a fork and add mayonnaise, Dijon mustard, paprika and tiny bacon pieces with Mix until creamy. Add salt and pepper to taste.
5. Stuff egg whites with the yolk-bacon mixture.
6. Dust deviled eggs with paprika and drizzle with fresh minced parsley.
Nutritional values (per serving)
Carbs – 1 g, protein – 25 g, fat – 41 g

52. Eggs Benedict With Avocado And Bacon Recipe

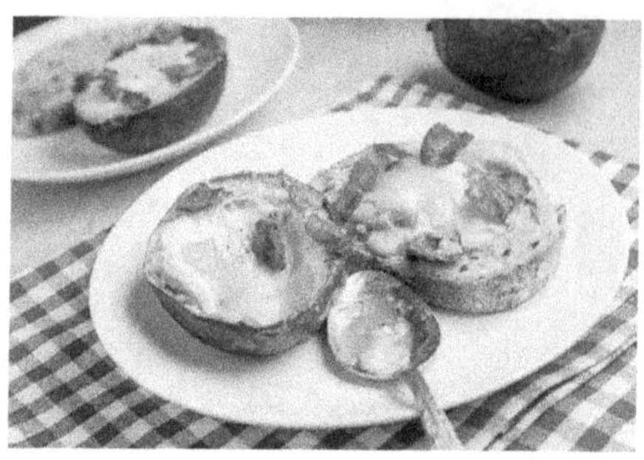

INGREDIENTS (for 2 servings)
Egg – 4 pcs
Cooked bacon slices – 4 pcs (cut in half)
Avocado – 1 piece
Apple cider vinegar – 15 ml
Fresh parsley
For Hollandaise Sauce
Melted ghee – 100 ml
Egg yolk – 2pcs
Lemon juice – 15 ml
Pinch of sea salt
Pinch of cayenne pepper

INSTRUCTIONS
1. Make the Hollandaise sauce: whisk egg yolks, 15 ml of lemon juice, a pinch of cayenne and salt.
2. Cook sauce using the steamer. Whisk constantly and pour in melted ghee. Cook until thicken.
3. Take a saucepan with water and pour 15 ml of apple cider vinegar. Bring to a boil. Slack the fire and break four eggs. Cook 3 minutes.
4. Line a dish with avocado slices, top with cooked bacon slices and poached eggs. Be sure to drizzle with Hollandaise sauce.
5. if desired, garnish with fresh parsley.
Nutritional values (per serving)
Carbs – 11 g, protein – 24 g, fat – 64 g

53. Simple Korean-Style Cucumbers Recipe

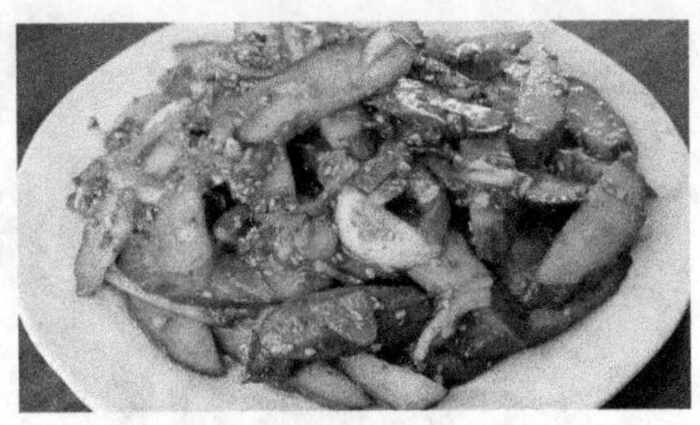

INGREDIENTS (for 2 servings)
English cucumber – 1
Coconut aminos – ¼ cup
White wine vinegar – 30 ml
Raw honey – 25 gr
Garlic bulbets – 1 piece
Fresh ginger – 25 gr
Red chili powder – 5gr
Green onion – 1piece
Sea salt, ground black pepper

INSTRUCTIONS
1. Combine in a bowl coconut aminos, white wine vinegar, raw honey, minced garlic and ginger, red chili powder, salt, pepper.
2. Slice cucumber and add to this mixture. Sprinkle with minced green onions.
3. Toss well.
4. Keep in the fridge before serving.
Nutritional values (per serving)
Carbs – 22 g, protein – 1 g, fat – 0 g

54. Simple Dill-Garlic Pickles Recipe

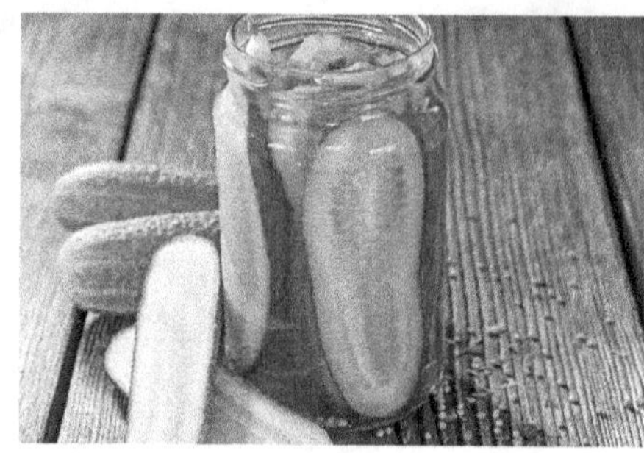

INGREDIENTS (for 4 servings)
 Cucumber – 1 piece
Water – 350 ml
Apple cider vinegar – 60 ml
Whole black peppercorns – 20 gr
Garlic bulbets – 5 pcs
Fresh dill
Red pepper flakes – 5gr
Juice from half of one lemon
Sea salt

INSTRUCTIONS
1. Make a marinade: combine in a bowl 350 ml of water, 60ml of apple cider vinegar, lemon juice and sea salt. Mix well until all ingredients are dissolved.
2. Take two jars and divide sliced cucumber, garlic, whole black peppercorn, fresh dill sprigs and red pepper flakes equally among them.
3. Pour marinade equally among both jars up to the top.
4. Cover jars, shake well to combine all ingredients and refrigerate.
5. Let marinate for 1-2 days. Store in the fridge.
Nutritional values (per serving)
Carbs – 6 g, protein – 0 g, fat – 0 g

55. Slow Cooker Buffalo Chicken Meatballs Recipe

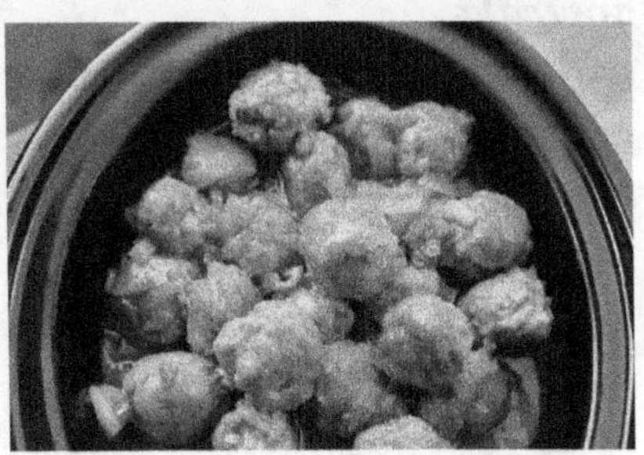

INGREDIENTS (for 4 servings)
Ground chicken – 450 gr
Almond meal – 28 gr
Egg – 1 piece
Garlic bulbets – 2 pcs
Green onions – 2 pcs
Buffalo sauce – 255 gr
Sea salt, ground black pepper

INSTRUCTIONS
1. Preheat your oven to 200 C. Mince garlic and cut green onions into thin slices.
2. Take a bowl, put there ground chicken, sliced green onion, minced garlic, almond meal, one egg. Add sea salt and black pepper to taste. Mix well.
3. Form meatballs. Place them onto a baking dish and cook for 5 minutes.
4. Switch off the oven and place chicken meatballs into a slow cooker. Pour in buffalo sauce, mix well.
5. Cook for 2 hours.
Nutritional values (per serving)
Carbs – 7 g, protein – 25 g, fat – 20 g

DESSERT RECIPES

56. Paleo Strawberry Shortcake

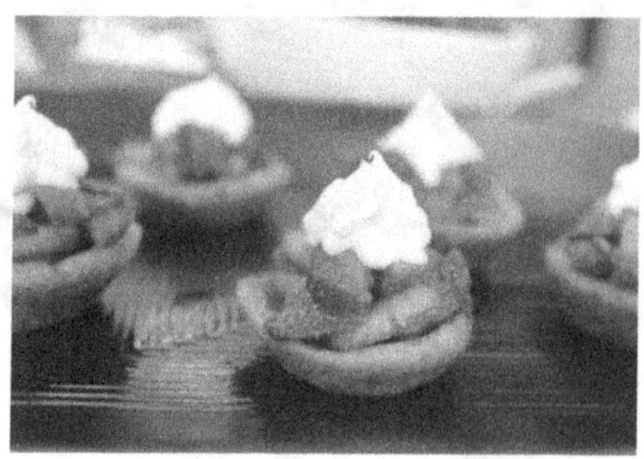

INGREDIENTS (for 8 servings)
For shortcake:
Almond flour – 375 gr
Egg – 2 pcs
Honey – 60 gr
Baking powder – 5 gr
Fresh strawberries – 2 cups
Sea salt – 1 gr
Lemon juice – 30 ml
For cream:
Full-cream coconut milk - 1 can
Honey – 30 gr
Vanilla extract – 5 gr

INSTRUCTIONS
1. Heat the oven to 160°C, take a parchment paper and line the whole baking sheet.
2. Combine eggs, honey and lemon juice. Beat up well.
3. Take a large bowl and combine dry ingredients. Make a well in the middle, and pour in egg mixture. Stir well until batter is ready
5. Drop the batter on the baking sheet with tablespoon and flatten a little.
6. Bake shortcakes for 15–20 minutes. Meanwhile, you can make coconut whipped cream.
7. Take 1 can of refrigerated full-cream coconut milk, open it, scoop the top layer of cream and put into a deep bowl. Loosen the waxy coconut with mixer and add 30 gr of honey and 5 gr of vanilla. Beat up until light and fluffy.
8. Remove shortcakes, let them cool for 3 minutes. Top each shortcake with sliced fresh strawberries and coconut whipped cream.
9. Serve and enjoy immediately!

Nutritional values (per 1 serving)
Carbs - 12 g, protein - 4 g, fat – 9 g, energy – 136 kcal

57. Paleo Buttermilk Pancakes

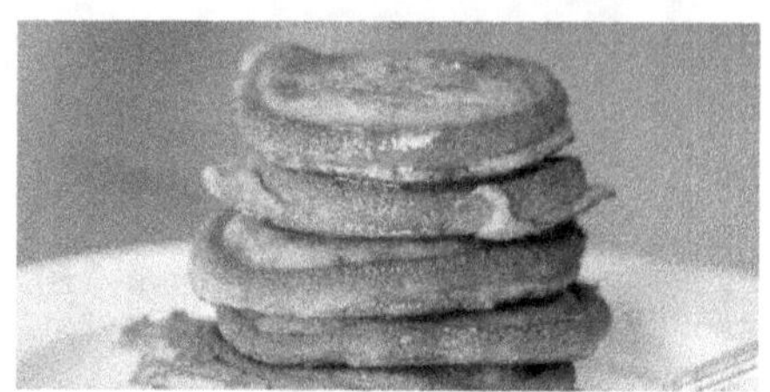

INGREDIENTS (for 8 pancakes)
Coconut flour - 45 gr
Almond flour - 45 gr
Egg – 3 pcs
Almond milk - 120 ml
Apple cider vinegar – 2 ml
Vanilla extract – 5 gr
Baking soda – 1 gr
Maple syrup – 10 ml
Butter - 25-30 gr
Sea salt

INSTRUCTIONS
1. Take a bowl and mix 120 ml of almond milk and 2 ml of apple cider vinegar. Set aside.
2. Take another separate large bowl and combine coconut flour, almond flour, eggs, almond milk and ½ teaspoon of vinegar mixture, vanilla extract, baking soda, erythritol, melted butter and a dash of sea salt. Mix all ingredients until smooth paste.
3. Heat greased griddle and pour the batter. Cook for 2-3 minutes on the one hand, then turn pancake and cook another 2 minutes on the other hand.
4. While preparing pancakes you may keep finished pancakes in the oven on separate dish. They will be warm.
5. When you finish remove warm pancakes and serve with any condiments you like.
Nutritional values (per 1 pancake)
Carbs - 5 g, protein – 3 g, fat – 6 g, fiber - 2 g, energy – 85 kcal

58. Paleo Salted Chocolate Caramel Bars

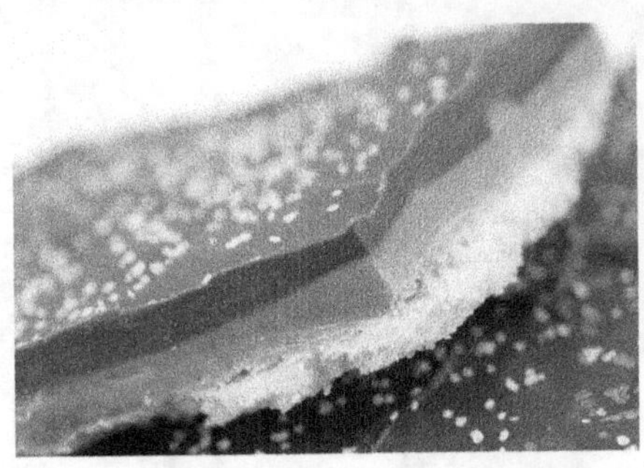

INGREDIENT (for 16 servings)
For Chocolate Layers
Raw cacao powder – 64 gr + 50 gr
Coconut oil – 120 ml
Pure maple syrup – 60 ml
For the Caramel Layer
Almond butter – 113 gr
Maple syrup – 120 ml
Coconut oil – 80 ml
Vanilla extract – 30 gr
Sea salt
For Garnishing
Sea salt

INSTRUCTION
1. Take a square pan ad grease it.
2. First of all make chocolate layers. Combine raw cacao powder coconut oil and maple syrup. Mix and let it completely melted.
3. Pour 2/3 chocolate mixture into the greased pan. Put the pan with chocolate mixture into the freezer for 15 minutes.
4. Take a small saucepan and combine all ingredients for caramel and heat it. Mix thoroughly until melted. Let it cool slightly.
5. Pour 2/3 of caramel over the cooled chocolate and spread on the chocolate layer.
6. Back in the fridge for 15-20 minutes.
7. Pour the remaining chocolate mixture over top, carefully smooth.
8. Then again return the pan and freeze to set for 30 minutes.
9. Slice ready bars into squares/ Keep n refrigerator.

Nutritional values (per serving)
Carbs -16, 4 g, protein – 3 g, fat – 17 g, energy – 221 kcal

59. Paleo Apple Pie Cheesecake

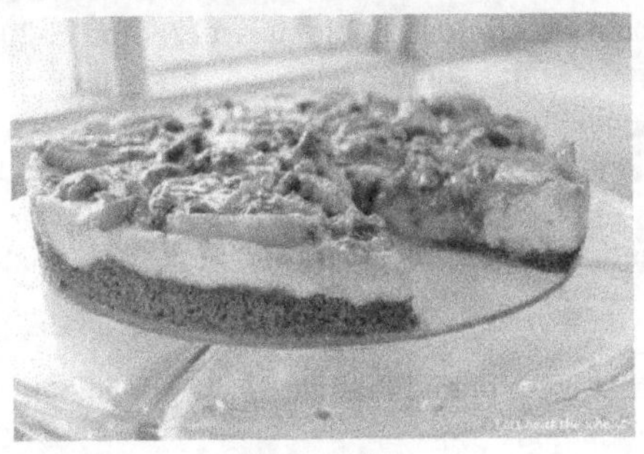

INGREDIENTS (for 12 servings)
<u>For Crust</u>
Almond flour – 140 gr
Vanilla extract – 10 gr
Coconut sugar – 95 gr
Palm shortening – 1/3 cup
<u>For Cheesecake</u>
Cashews - 2 ½ cup
Vanilla extract – 10 gr
Lemon juice – 5 ml
Coconut milk – 54 ml
<u>For Caramel</u>
Honey – 320 gr
Coconut sugar – 48 gr
Vanilla extract – 10 gr
Coconut milk – 80 ml
<u>For Topping</u>
Apple – 4pcs
Cinnamon – 20 gr
Water – 40 ml
Pecan pieces – 1/3 cup

INSTRUCTION
1. Preheat your oven to 175 degrees. Prepare crust: take a stand up mixer, combine all crust ingredients in it. Blend until it looks crumbly. Transfer this mixture into a pan. Bake for twenty minutes or until golden brown. Take ready crust out of the oven. Let cool.

2. Make topping: wash, dry and then peel apples. Cut them into quarters, put on the dish, pour water and add the cinnamon. Mix these ingredients and place in the heated oven. Cook fifteen minutes.

3. Meanwhile, you can prepare filling for cheesecake. Drain and rinse cashews, pour them into a blender and add vanilla, lemon juice and coconut milk. Blend all these ingredients (NOTE cashews must be fully grounded). Cashew mixture is ready. Pour it on top of cooled crust. Put in the freezer for 15-20 minutes.

4. When apples are done, drain the water and set aside.

5. Now make the caramel: combine honey, coconut sugar, vanilla extract, coconut milk in a big saucepan. Turn on the oven and bring to a boil. Cook on medium fire for 7-10 minutes until this mixture get thick. Then cool caramel for five minutes.

6. Take the pan out of the freezer and put apples on top of cashew mixture and pour the caramel. Sprinkle with pecan pieces.

7. Put into freezer for 2 hours.

8. Cooled Paleo Apple Pie Cheesecake is ready! Cut into 12 pieces. Enjoy!

Nutritional values (per serving)

Carbs -54 g, protein – 6 g, fat – 24 g, energy – 430kcal

60. Paleo Strawberry Ginger Crisp

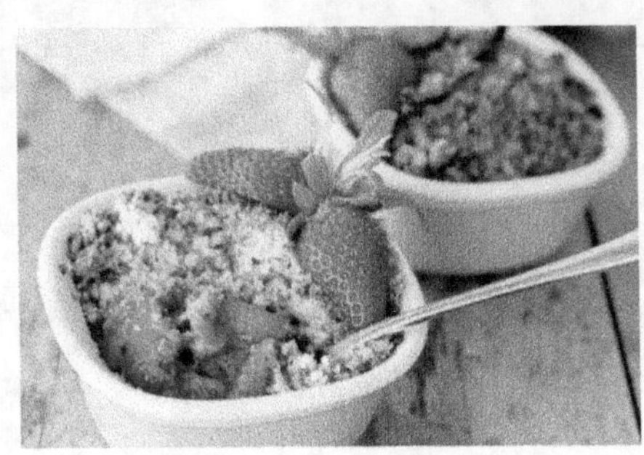

INGREDIENTS (for 4 servings)
For the filling
Chopped strawberries – 3 cups
Freshly grated ginger – 25 gr
Zest of one lemon
Lemon juice – 18 ml
Chia seeds – 25 gr
Maple syrup – 50-60 gr
Tapioca starch – 50 gr
Salt – 5 gr
For the topping
Almond flour – 70 gr
Cashew flour – 25 gr
Coconut flour – 25 gr
Chopped walnuts – 40 gr
Cinnamon – 5 gr
Maple syrup – 20 gr
Coconut oil – 15 ml
Salt – 2 gr

INSTRUCTION
1. Preheat oven to 175 C. Grease baking dish with oil.
2. Combine in a bowl all ingredients for filing: 3 cups of chopped strawberries,25 gr of freshly grated ginger, zest, 18 ml of lemon juice, 25gr of chia seeds, 50 gr of maple syrup, 50 gr of tapioca starch and salt. Toss together.
3. Combine in a separate bowl all ingredients for topping: 70 gr of almond flour, 25 gr of cashew flour, 25 gr of coconut flour, 40 gr of chopped walnuts, 5 gr of cinnamon, 20 gr of maple syrup, and salt. Mix together. Add 15 ml of coconut oil and continue to mix until it becomes a crumbly texture.

4. Pour this filling into the greased baking dish. Drizzle the topping and bake for twenty minutes.
5. After 20 minutes remove the dish from the oven, cool for a few minutes.
6. Serve warm.
Nutritional values (per serving)
Carbs - 25 g, protein – 7 g, fat – 15 g, energy – 247 kcal

61. Pumpkin Chocolate Chip Cookies

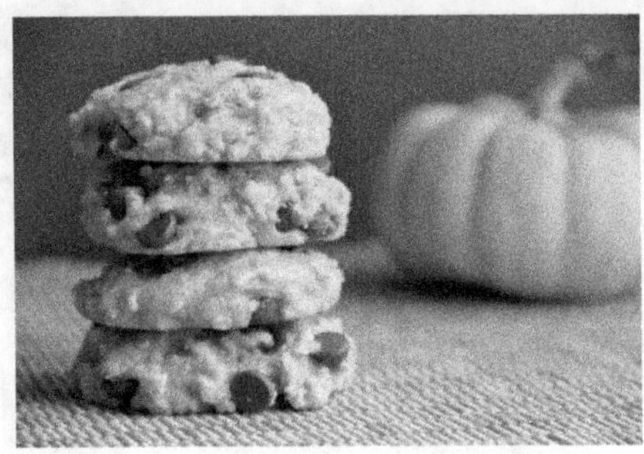

INGREDIENTS (for 24 servings)
Butter – 76 gr)
Pumpkin puree – 80 gr
Maple syrup – 113 gr
Egg – 1 piece
Pure vanilla extract – 10 gr
Tapioca flour – 85 gr
Coconut flour – 45 gr
Pumpkin pie spice- 10 gr
Baking soda – 5 gr
Chocolate chips – 30 gr
Sea salt

INSTRUCTION
1. Melt butter and stir in 80 gr of pumpkin puree, 113 gr of maple syrup, one egg and 10 gr of vanilla extract. Mix.
2. Stir in 85 gr of tapioca flour,45 gr of coconut flour,10 gr of pumpkin pie spice, 5 gr of baking soda and salt. Mix once again and put 30 gr of chocolate chips. Mix carefully.
3. Put batter into the fridge for half an hour.
4. Meanwhile, switch on the oven and preheat it to 190 C.
5. Prepare baking dish, line it with parchment. Turn cool batter on the dish with spoon and flatten each cookie.
6. Bake pumpkin chocolate chip cookies for 12-15 minutes. Enjoy!
Nutritional values (per serving)
Carbs - 6 g, protein – 1 g, fat – 4 g, energy – 57 kcal

62. Paleo Banana Pudding

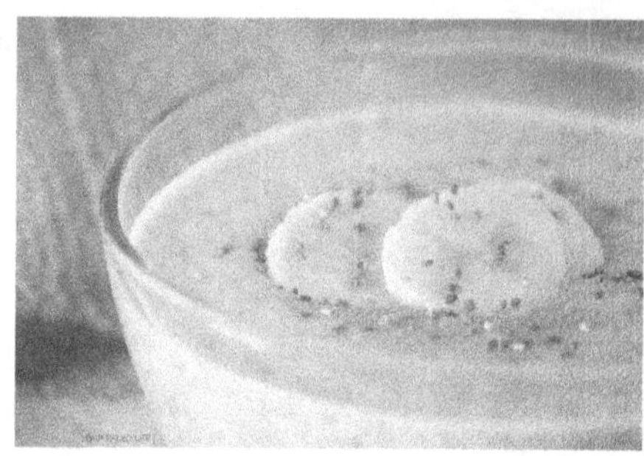

INGREDIENTS (for 4 servings)
Egg yolks – 4 pcs
Honey – 85 gr
Arrowroot powder – 35 gr
Banana – 2 pcs (mashed)
Banana – 1 piece (sliced)
Whole coconut milk – 480 ml
Vanilla extract – 10 gr
Salt
Walnuts

INSTRUCTION
1. Beat together 4 egg yolks, honey, arrowroot powder. Set aside.
2. Pour coconut milk into the saucepan and warm up. After 5 minutes pour warm coconut milk into the egg mixture. Mix constantly. Pour egg-milk mixture back into the saucepan. Cook 2-3 minutes until thickened. (NOTE This mixture shouldn't boil!)
3. Pour over the mixture into a bowl and add in the vanilla extract and two mashed bananas. Transfer into the fridge. Let chill for one hour.
4. Serve pudding in glasses topped with banana slices and crushed walnuts.
5. Serve immediately!
Nutritional values (per serving)
Carbs - 50 g, protein – 6 g, fat – 29 g, energy – 471 kcal

63. TURMERIC GOLDEN MILK POPSICLES

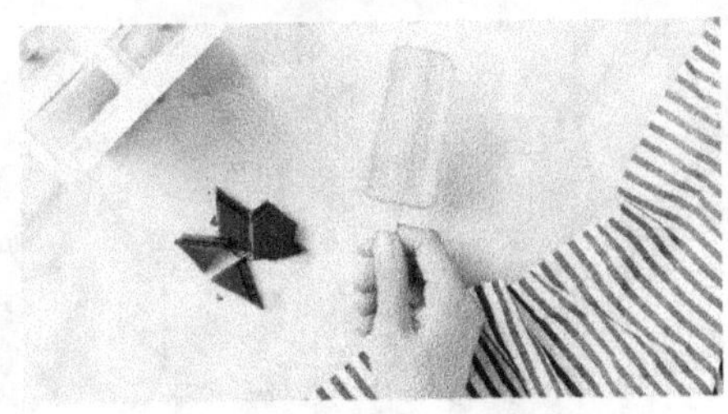

INGREDIENTS (for 6 servings)
Light canned coconut milk – 480 ml
Honey – 90 gr
Ground turmeric – 10 gr
Ground ginger – 10 gr
A dash of freshly ground black pepper

INSTRUCTION
1. Take a blender and combine all ingredients in a blender bowl. Blend until smooth.
2. Pour turmeric golden milk mixture into popsicle molds and place in the freeze for 1 hour. Insert colorful sticks.
Freeze for 4 hours.
Nutritional values (per 1 popsicle)
Carbs – 10 g, protein – 0,1 g, fat – 4,5 g, energy – 84 kcal

64. Dark Chocolate Nut Clusters with Sea Salt

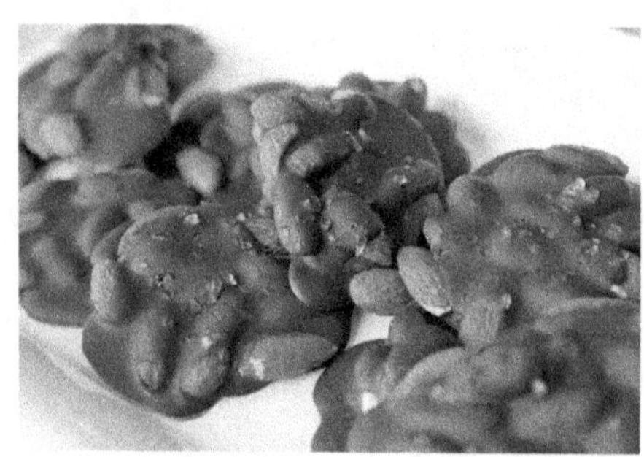

INGREDIENTS (for 20 clusters)
Almonds - 20 pcs
Pecan halves – 20 pcs
Walnut halves – 20 pcs
Ghirardelli Dark Chocolate Melting Wafers – 1 package
Sea salt

INSTRUCTION
1. Melt chocolate.
2. Dip walnut into the melted chocolate and then transfer to a piece of wax paper. Dip pecan and put on the top of the walnut and finish with almond. Form cluster. So do the same with remaining nuts.
3. Sprinkle each cluster with sea salt. Enjoy!!
Nutritional values (per one cluster)
Carbs – 3 g, protein – 1 g, fat – 5 g, energy – 54 kcal

65. CRANBERRY PEAR SAUCE

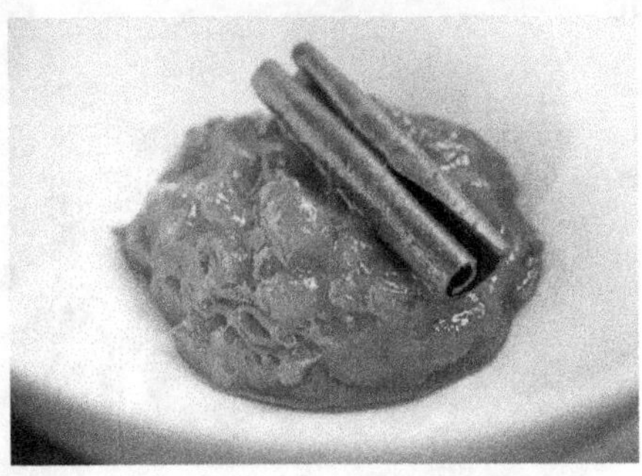

INGREDIENTS (for 13)
Fresh cranberries – 340 gr
Pear – 2 pcs   s, peeled and cored, cubed small
Raw honey – 170 gr
Water – 240 ml

INSTRUCTION
1. Peel and core pears, cut on small cubes.
2. Combine all ingredients in a saucepan and bring to a boil. Slack the fire and simmer 15 min until sauce thickens.
3. Turn off the oven, empty sauce into deep bowl and let it cool. Serve!
Nutritional values (per 1/4 cup)
Carbs – 16 g, protein – 0 g, fat – 0 g, energy – 61 kcal

PALEO SALADS

66. Paleo Broccoli Salad

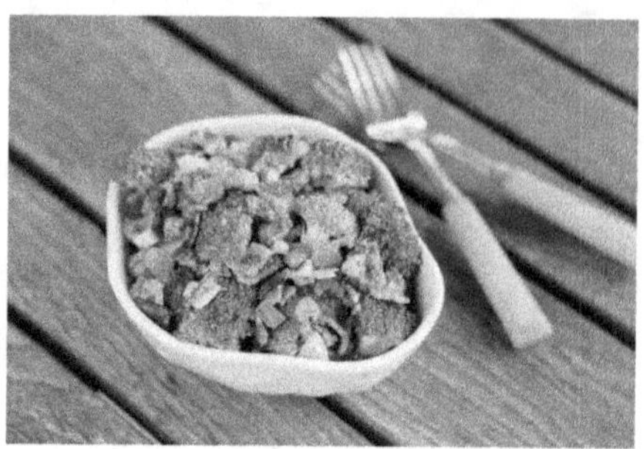

INGREDIENTS (for 4 servings)
Paleo mayonnaise – 227 gr
Honey – 60 gr
Balsamic vinegar – 30 ml
Broccoli curds – 4 cups
Dried raisins – 65 gr
Slivered almonds – 65 gr
Red onions – 1 piece

INSTRUCTION
1. Firstly make dressing for your salad combining your favorite ingredients: honey, paleo mayonnaise and balsamic vinegar.
2. Prepare a deep bowl with ice water. Set aside.
3. Mix water and salt in a bowl. Pour salted water in the pan and bring to a boil. Add broccoli curds and cook for 1 minute, then, after boiling the broccoli, submerge it in ice water to stop the cooking process. Dry cooked broccoli curds using paper towels and slice into bite-size pieces. Put these pieces in a separate serving dish.
4. Add dried raisins, slivered almonds, sliced red onion to broccoli. Pour the dressing and mix well. Cool for one hour.
5. Enjoy cold!
Nutritional values (per 1 serving)
Carbs - 40 g, protein - 6 g, fat – 20 g, energy – 340 kcal

67. Cranberry Avocado Salad

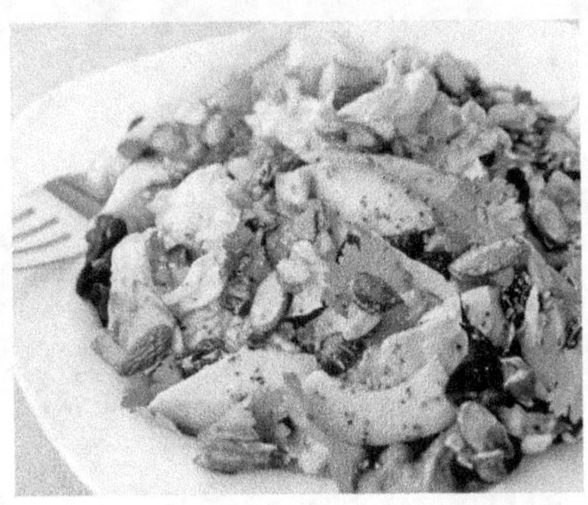

INGREDIENTS (for 4 servings)
Baby mixed greens (spinach, arugula)- 340 gr
Avocado – 2 pcs
Dried cranberries – ¾ cup
Roasted almonds – ¾ cup
<u>For the dressing</u>
Extra virgin olive oil – 2/3 cup
Poppy seeds – 25-30 gr
Paprika – 2-3 gr
Dried mustard – 10 gr
Minced sweet onion – 30 gr
White balsamic vinegar – 60 ml
Raw honey (optional) – ¼ cup
Sea salt
Ground black pepper

INSTRUCTION
1. First make dressing for our salad. In a separate bowl combine all ingredients for the dressing. Salt and pepper to taste. Mix well.
2. Put greens in the bottom of a large bowl. Slice avocado and add dried cranberries.
3. Pour a quarter of the dressing on the top. Mix gently.
4. Spread roasted almonds over the salad.
5. Add dressing if you like. Enjoy!
Nutritional values (per serving)
Carbs - 24 g, protein – 7 g, fat – 40 g, energy – 461 kcal

68. AHI TUNA WATERMELON SALAD

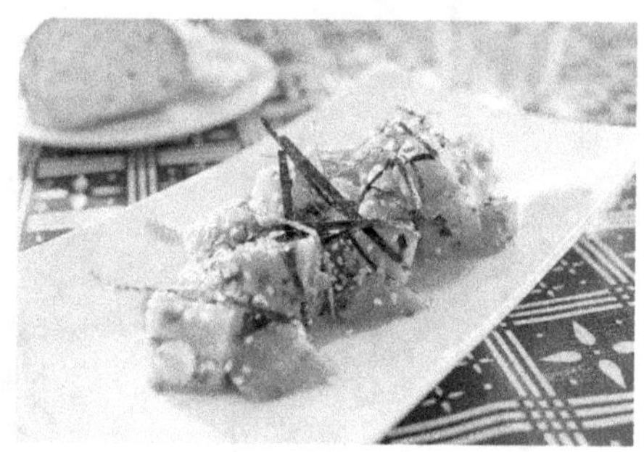

INGREDIENTS (4 servings)
Tuna fillet – 450 gr
Coconut aminos – 35 ml
Fresh lime juice – 35 ml
Grapeseed oil – 15ml
Sesame oil – 15 ml
Honey – 25 gr
A dash of fresh minced ginger
Minced garlic – 10 gr
A dash of red pepper flakes
Watermelon – 2 cups , half-inch cubes
Persian cucumber – 1 piece , sliced 1/8-inch thick with mandolin, rolled tight
Finely sliced shallot – 1 piece
Cilantro

INSTRUCTION
1. Take fillets and trim away any skin. Cut tuna fillets into small cubes. Put in a bowl.
2. Take another dish and whisk together coconut aminos, fresh lime juice, grapeseed oil and sesame oil, honey, minced garlic, fresh minced ginger and red pepper flakes.
3. Pour this sauce over tuna cubes and salt at the end. Transfer in the fridge and leave to marinate for an hour.
4. Meanwhile, cut watermelon into cubes and slice cucumber. Rolled them.
5. After an hour, divide marinated tuna into 4 plates. Garnish with watermelon cubes and cucumber rolls, drizzle with finely sliced shallots and cilantro.
Nutritional values (serving size ¼)
Carbs – 13 g, protein – 29,5 g, fat – 5,5 g, energy – 217 kcal

69. BREAKFAST BLT SALAD

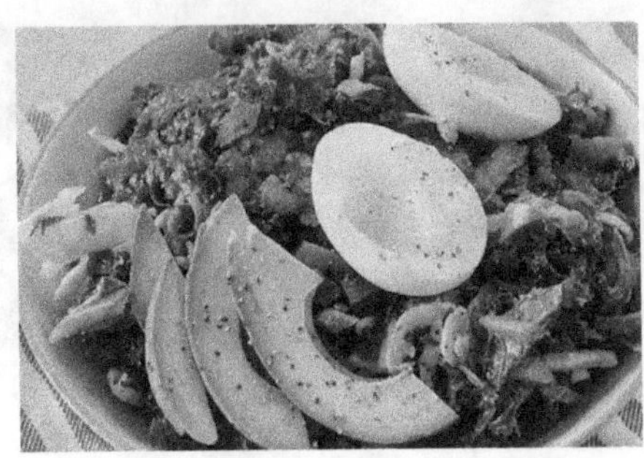

INGREDIENTS (for 2 servings)
Eggs – 2 pcs
Shredded Lacinto kale – 3 cups
Red wine vinegar – 5 ml
Extra virgin olive oil – 10 ml
Kosher salt, black pepper
Chopped bacon – 4 slices
Avocado – 55 gr (sliced)
Grape tomatoes 10 pcs

INSTRUCTION
1. Make some preparations: cook eggs, slice avocado, chop bacon, cut grape tomatoes into halves and shred kale.
2. When preparations are done, take a bowl and combine shredded kale, olive oil, red wine vinegar and salt. Bruise kale with your hands until it softens.
3. Divide juicy kale between two bowls, add chopped bacon, tomatoes halves, avocado slices and cutted eggs. Salt and pepper to taste.
4. Mmmm! Yummy!
Nutritional values (per 1 salad)
Carbs – 18 g, protein – 17,5 g, fat – 18 g, energy – 292 kcal

70. Asparagus Egg and Bacon Salad with Dijon Vinaigrette

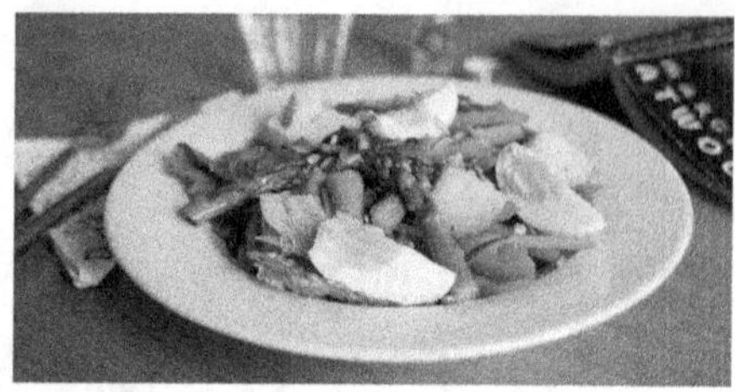

INGREDIENTS (for 1 serving)
Boiled egg – 1 piece
Chopped asparagus – 1 2/3 cup
Cooked bacon – 2 slices
Dijon mustard - 5 gr
Extra virgin olive oil – 5 ml
Red wine vinegar – 5 ml
Salt, pepper

INSTRUCTION
1. Put asparagus in a saucepan with boiled water and cook 2-3 minutes. Drain and rinse in cold water. Set aside.
2. Take a small bowl and combine Dijon mustard, olive oil, red wine vinegar, salt and pepper. Slice boiled egg on the plate.
3. Spread asparagus on the pattern, add egg slices and bacon. Sprinkle with vinaigrette. Enjoy!
Nutritional values (per 1 salad)
Carbs – 11 g, protein – 16 g, fat – 13 g, energy – 219 kcal

71. Shredded Raw Brussels Sprout Salad with Bacon and Avocado

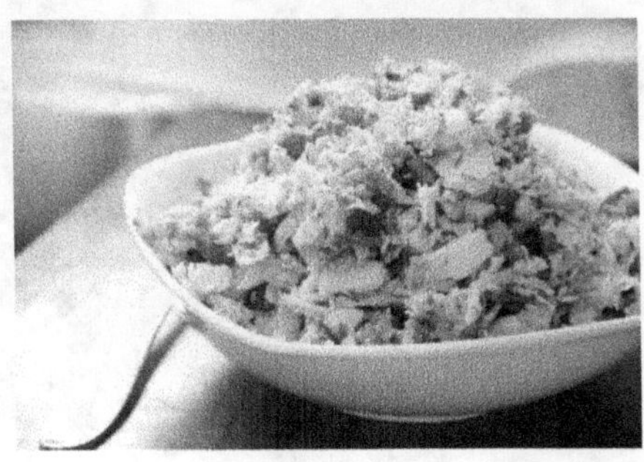

INGREDIENTS (for 2 servings)
Bacon – 3 slices
Shredded brussels sprouts – 3 cups
Avocado – 1 (115 gr)
For the vinaigrette
Dijon mustard - 5 gr
Olive oil – 20 ml
Red wine vinegar – 30 ml +5 ml
Chopped red onion – 50 gr
Kosher salt

INSTRUCTION
1. Dice bacon slices and fry until crispy. Drain using a paper towel. Put on the plate.
2. Make vinaigrette: combine all ingredients according to the recipe. Whisk well.
3. Place shredded Brussels sprouts in a bowl, pour in vinaigrette and top with diced avocado and bacon crisps.
4. Enjoy immediately!
Nutritional values (per 2 cups)
Carbs – 18,5 g, protein –10 g, fat – 21 g, energy – 284 kcal

72. Spiralized Carrot Salad with Lemon and Dijon

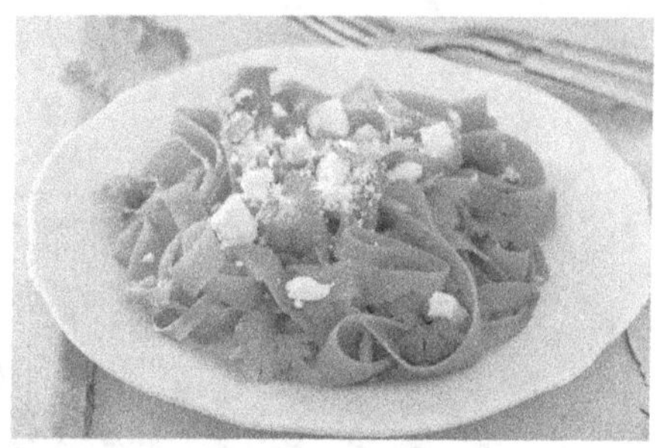

INGREDIENTS (for 4 servings)
Carrot – 450 gr
Dijon mustard – 30 g
Just squeezed lemon juice of one lemon
Extra virgin olive oil – 15 ml
Kosher salt
Ground black pepper
Chopped shallots – 15 gr

INSTRUCTIONS
1. Peel and spiralize carrots.
2. Make dressing: combine together all ingredients. Toss well.
3. Add carrot noodles and toss well again. Cool and enjoy!
Nutritional values (per 1cup)
Carbs – 12 g, protein –1 g, fat – 4 g, energy – 84 kcal

73. LOBSTER ASPARAGUS CHOPPED SALAD

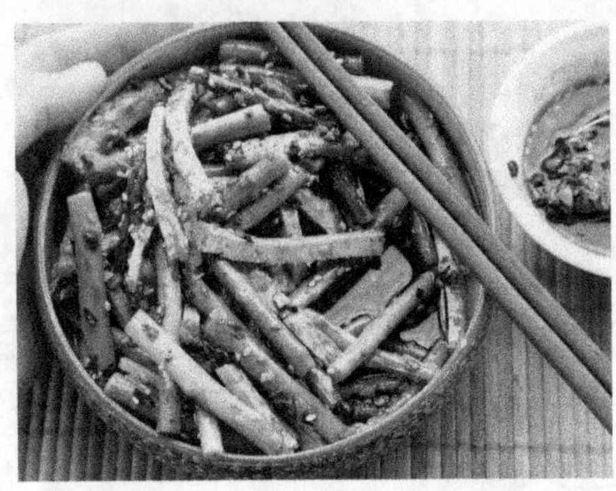

INGREDIENTS (for 2 servings)
Cooked lobster – 225 gr
Chopped asparagus – 3 ½ cup
Extra virgin olive oil – 20 ml
Fresh lemon juice – 30 ml
Cherry tomatoes – ½ cup
Diced red onion – 50 gr
Chopped basil leaf – 1 piece
Kosher salt
Black pepper

INSTRUCTIONS
1. Chop cooked lobster, cut tomatoes into quarters, dice red onion, chop asparagus.
2. Take a saucepan, pour in water and bring to a boil. Put chopped asparagus and cook 2-3 minutes.
3. Drain asparagus and rinse in cold water. Lay aside.
4. Take a small bowl and mix together olive oil, fresh lemon juice, add salt and pepper.
5. Its time to combine all ingredients. Asparagus, chopped lobster, cherry tomatoes, diced red onion, chopped basil leaves and sauce.
Nutritional values (per 1 salad)
Carbs – 14 g, protein – 27 g, fat – 10,5 g, energy – 247 kcal

74. AVOCADO AND LUMP CRAB SALAD

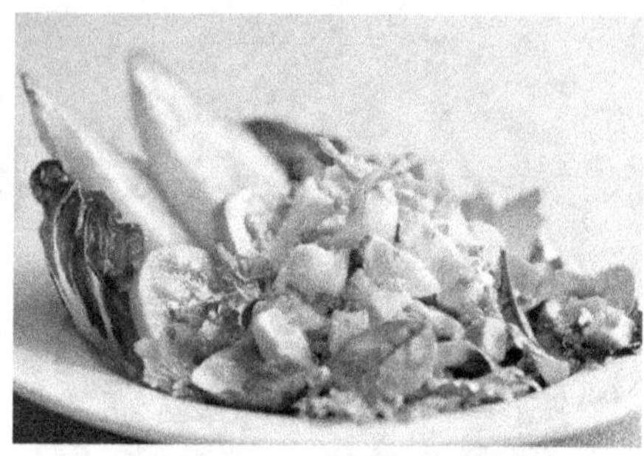

INGREDIENTS (for 2 servings)
Hass avocado – 1 piece (140 gr)
Lump crab meat – 45 gr
Chopped red onion – 50 gr
Fresh lime juice – 25 ml
Chopped fresh cilantro – 25 gr
Grape tomatoes – 2 pcs
Olive oil – 3 ml
Salt, black pepper
Butter lettuce leaves – 2 pcs

INSTRUCTIONS
1. Chop red onion and dice grape tomatoes. Peel avocado, cut in halves and scoop the pulp.
2. Combine in one large bowl crab meat, chopped onion, fresh lime juice, diced tomatoes, chopped fresh cilantro, olive oil. Salt and pepper to taste. Toss carefully.
3. Take avocado halves, drizzle with salt and stuff with crab salad.
4. You will get two servings, two stuffed avocado halves.
5. Put butter lettuce leaves on two plates and place stuffed avocado in the center.
Nutritional values (per 1 stuffed avocado half)
Carbs – 9 g, protein –9,5 g, fat – 13 g, energy – 178 kcal

75. Raw Kale Caesar Salad

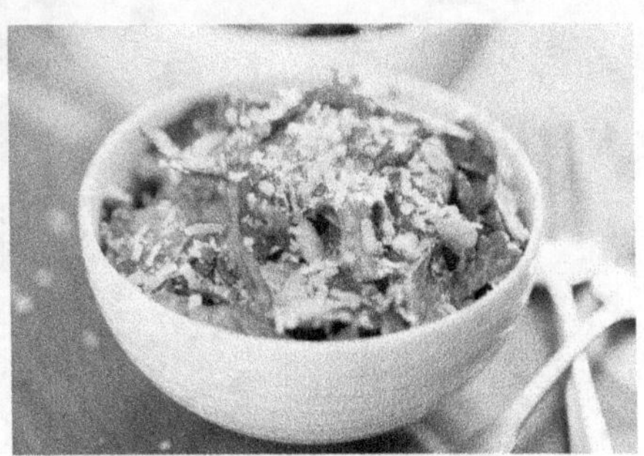

INGREDIENTS
Balanced Babe Cashew Caesar dressing – 120 gr
Dinosaur kale – 1 bunch
Nutritional yeast – 35 gr

INSTRUCTIONS
1. Wash and dry kale and dressing.
2. Mix in a bowl. Sprinkle with nutritional yeast. Enjoy!
Nutritional values (per serving)
Carbs – 22.1 g, protein –8,6 g, fat – 43,5 g, energy – 510 kcal

76. Roasted Vegetable Salad With Cilantro Dressing Recipe

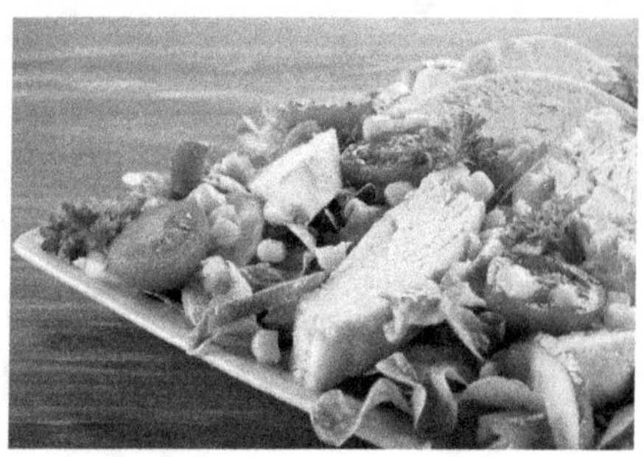

INGREDIENTS (for 4 servings)
Zucchini – 1 piece
Aubergine – 1 piece
Onion – 1 piece
Bell pepper – 1piece
Mixed greens – 7 cups
Olive oil – 45 ml;
Fresh lime juice – 30 ml
Cumin – 5 gr
Sea salt, ground black pepper
 For the Cilantro Dressing
Fresh cilantro leaves – 1 cup
Almond milk – 120 ml
Water – 60 ml
Garlic bulbets – 2 pcs
Juice and zest of one lime
Sea salt, ground black pepper

INSTRUCTIONS
1. Heat the oven to 190 C.
2. Prepare a bowl and mix sliced zucchini, diced aubergine, onion, bell pepper, olive oil, fresh lime juice, cumin, salt, pepper. Toss well.
3. Grease your baking tray, place veggies and roast 20 minutes.
4. Meanwhile, make cilantro dressing. Combine all necessary ingredients in a blender. Pulse until smooth. Add salt and pepper.
5. Place 7 cups of mixed greens in a bowl, put roasted vegetables on the top, pour cilantro dressing. Toss.
Nutritional values (per serving)

Carbs – 14 g, protein – 4 g, fat – 11 g

PALEO BEVERAGES

77. Melon with Kiwi and Mango Smoothie

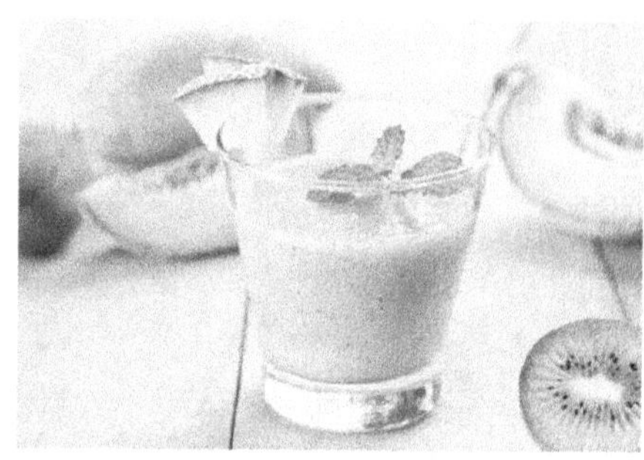

INGREDIENTS (for 4 Servings)
Kiwi – 2 pcs
Melon – 1 x 170 gr
Mango – 1 piece
Water – 240 ml

INSTRUCTIONS
1. Make preparations: peel and slice kiwis, cut melon into chunks and cut mango into chunks.
2. Put ingredients into blender bowl and blend until smooth.
3. Garnish with mint leaves.
Nutritional values (per serving)
Carbs – 64,19 g, protein – 4,12 g, fat – 1,55 g, energy – 259 kcal

78. Antioxidant Berry Shake

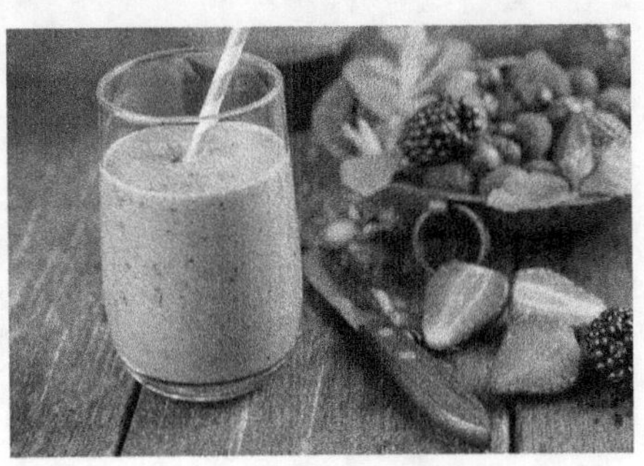

INGREDIENTS (for 1 serving)
Coconut milk - 120 ml
Cold water – 60 ml
Frozen banana – ½
Frozen raspberries – 70 gr
Frozen blueberries – 70 gr
Chia seeds – 25 gr

INSTRUCTIONS
1. Take a bowl and put there all ingredients.
2. Blend until smooth. Serve!

79. Orange, Mango and Kiwi Smoothie Recipe

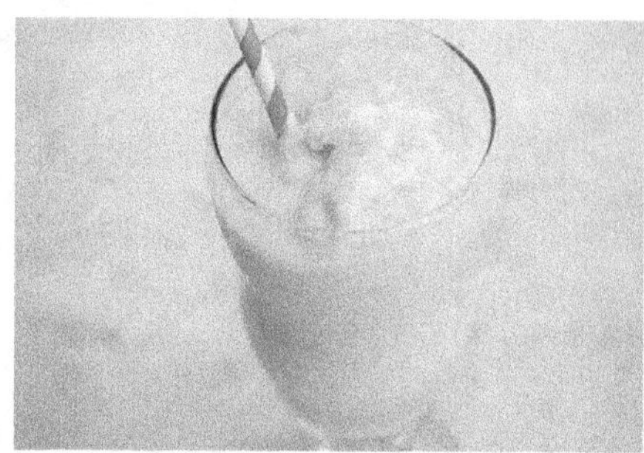

INGREDIENTS (for 2 servings)
Kiwi – 2 pcs
Juice of two or three oranges
Mango – 1 piece
Fresh lemon juice – 30ml
Fresh ginger – 15 gr
Fresh fruit slices

INSTRUCTIONS
1. Mince fresh ginger. Peel mango, kiwis and cut fruits into big chunks. Put them in a blender.
2. Pour in fresh orange and lemon juices, minced ginger.
3. Blend until smooth.
4. Divide into 2 glasses, garnish with fresh fruit slices.
Nutritional values (per 2 servings)
Carbs – 73 g, protein – 4 g, fat – 2 g

80. Carrot And Beet Juice Recipe

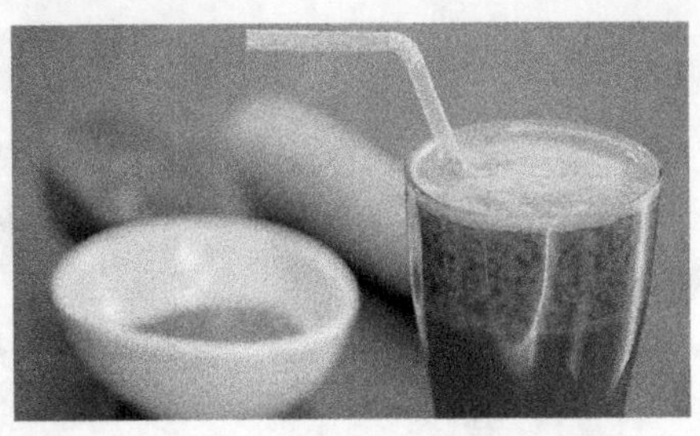

INGREDIENTS (for 2 servings)
Beet – 2 pcs
Carrot – 2 pcs
Granny Smith apple – 1 piece
Celery stalk – 1 piece
Tomato – 1 piece
Water - 120 ml
Half of one cucumber
Fresh lime juice – 30 ml

INSTRUCTIONS
1. Peel beets, carrots, apple and cucumber.
2. Put all ingredients in a blender. Pulse until smooth.
3. Serve cold.
Nutritional values (per 2 servings)
Carbs – 35 g, protein – 4 g, fat – 1 g

81. Pumpkin Banana Smoothie Recipe

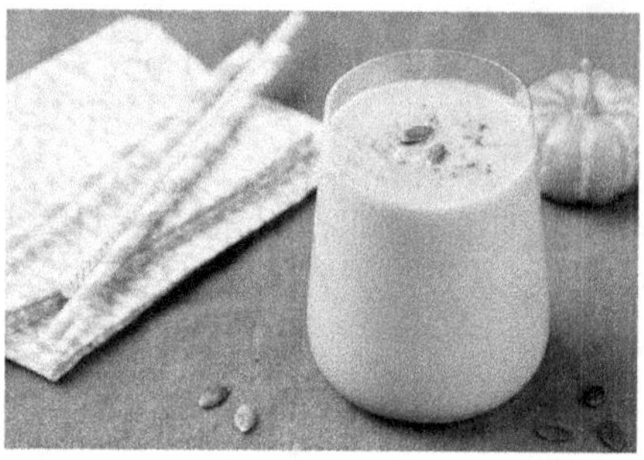

INGREDIENTS (for 1 serving)
Pumpkin puree – 100 ml
Banana – 1 piece
Almond milk – 60 ml
Pumpkin pie spice – 2 gr
Ice cubes – 4-5 pcs

INSTRUCTIONS
1. Combine In a blender first four ingredients. Blend until smooth.
2. Add ice cubes and continue to blend.
3. Serve cold!
Nutritional values (per serving)
Carbs – 40 g, protein – 2 g, fat – 2 g

82. Traditional Red Sangria Recipe

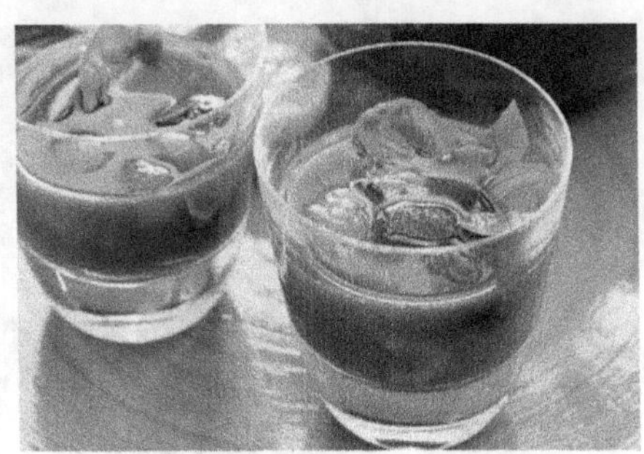

INGREDIENTS (for 4 servings)
Spanish red wine – 1 bottle
Apple juice – 240 ml
Orange juice – 240 ml
Lemon – 1 piece
Lime – 1 piece
Orange – 1 piece
Apple – 1 piece
Blueberries – ¼ cup
Raspberries – ¼ cup
Ice cubes

INSTRUCTIONS
1. Cut fruits into thin slices. Put them and on the bottom of a large glass pitcher.
2. Pour in liquids.
3. Add in ice cubes. Stir carefully and serve!

83. Spinach-Blueberry Frozen Smoothie Recipe

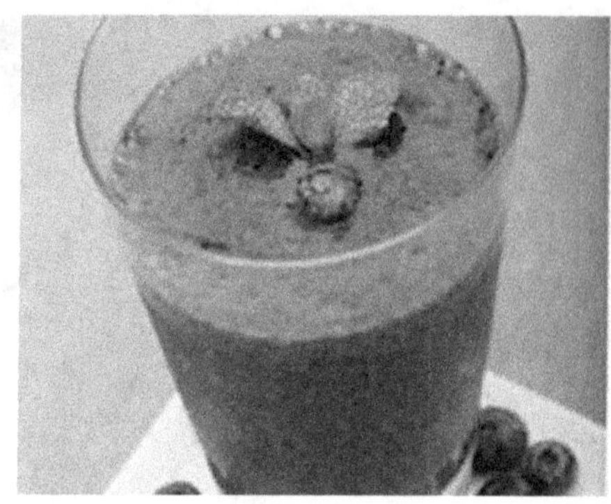

INGREDIENTS (for 2 servings)
Almond milk – 120 ml
Frozen blueberries – 2/3 cup
Spinach leaves – 1 cup
Frozen banana – 1 piece
Almond butter – 50 gr
Water – 120 ml

INSTRUCTIONS
1. Combine all smoothie ingredients in a blender. Blend until smooth.
2. Enjoy immediately!

84. Citrus and Watermelon Flavored Water Recipe

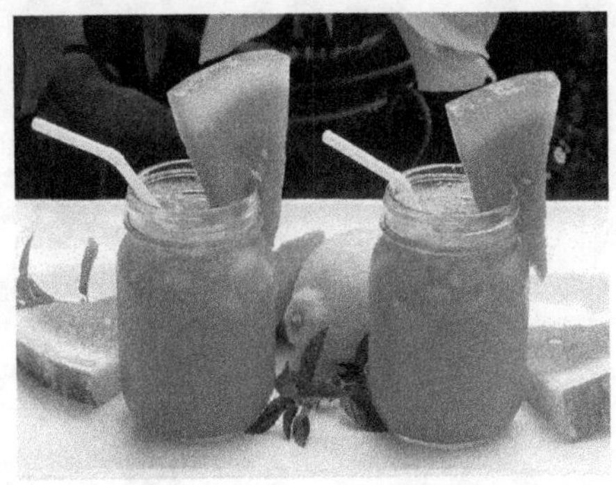

INGREDIENTS (for 4 servings)
Lime – 2pcs
Lemon – 1 piece
Watermelon – 2 cups
Red grapefruit – 1 piece
Cucumber – 1piece
Cold water

INSTRUCTIONS
1. Slice all fruits. Put them in the glass jug.
2. Pour in cold water.
3. Keep in fridge for several hours.
4. Enjoy this flavored drink!
Nutritional values (per serving)
Carbs – 17 g, protein – 1 g, fat – 1 g

85. Ginger Turmeric Orange Juice Recipe

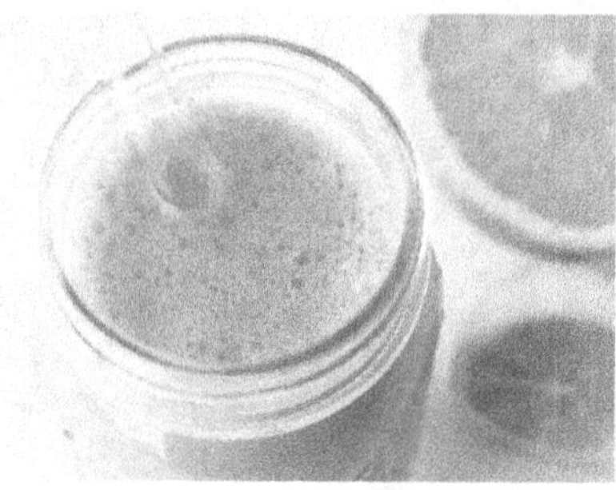

INGREDIENTS (for 4 servings)
Apple – 2 pcs
Orange – 4 pcs
Lemon – 1 piece
Fresh ginger – 25 gr
Fresh turmeric – 25 gr
Water – 240 ml

INSTRUCTIONS
1. Peel fruits. Chop apple, mince ginger and turmeric.
2. Put peeled fruits in a blender and blend until smooth.
3. Add minced spices and blend once again.
4. Pour in 240 ml of water and blend until you get a smooth juice
Nutritional values (per serving)
Carbs – 28 g, protein – 2 g, fat – 0 g

86. Cucumber, Parsley, Pineapple and Lemon Smoothie

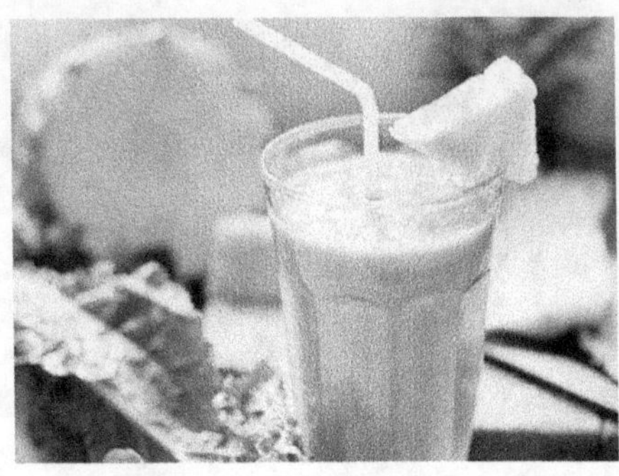

INGREDIENTS (for 2 smoothies)
Coconut water – 180 ml
Half of English cucumber
Parsley leaves – 1 bunch
Lemon – 2 pcs
Fresh pineapple – 280 gr
Liquid stevia – 5 drops

INSTRUCTIONS
1. Peel lemons, remove seeds and chop. Chop parsley leaves and pineapple.
2. Place all smoothie ingredients in a bowl and blend until smooth and creamy.
3. Pour into glasses.
Nutritional values (per 1 smoothie)
Carbs – 31 g, protein –2 g, fat – 0 g, energy – 118 kcal

87. Lemon, Ginger and Basil Iced Tea

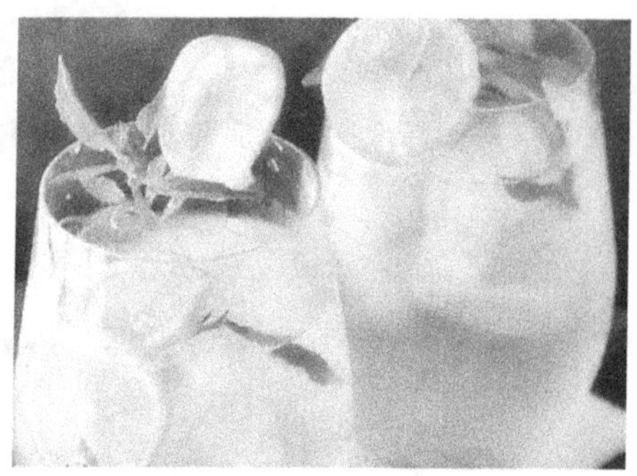

INGREDIENTS
Lemon – 2 pcs
 Ginger coins – 5 pcs
Basil leaves – 100 gr
Honey – 75 gr
Boiling water – 2,2 l

INSTRUCTIONS
1. Cut lemons into halves and put them into the jug, add five ginger coins and basil leaves.
2. Pour in boiling water and add honey. Steep tea.
3. When the tea reaches room temperature, take ginger coins, basil leaves and lemon halves out.
4. Better drink cool

88. Watermelon Agua Fresca

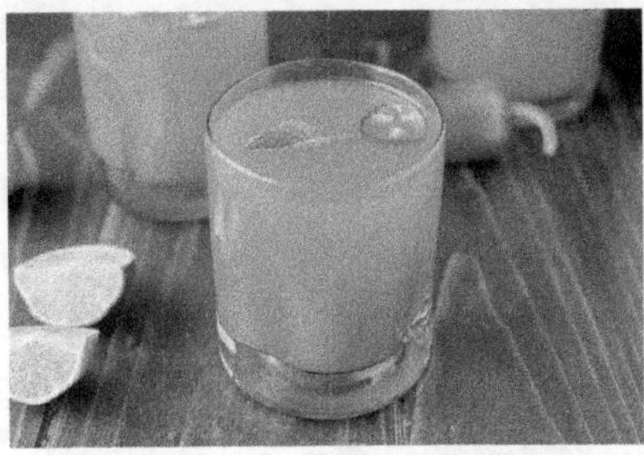

INGREDIENTS (for 4 servings)
Watermelon – 6 cups
Water – 180 ml
Lime slices – 4 pcs
Sprigs mint
Ice

INSTRUCTIONS
1. Take a melon, wash and dry. Cut in half, scoop seeds and cut into cubes.
2. Blend water and watermelon cubes. Blend until smooth.
3. Pour into glasses and garnish with sprigs mint and thin lime slices. If desired, add ice!
Nutritional values (per 1 cup)
Carbs – 16,5 g, protein –1,5 g, fat – 1 g, energy – 73 kcal

89. Matcha Green Tea Shots

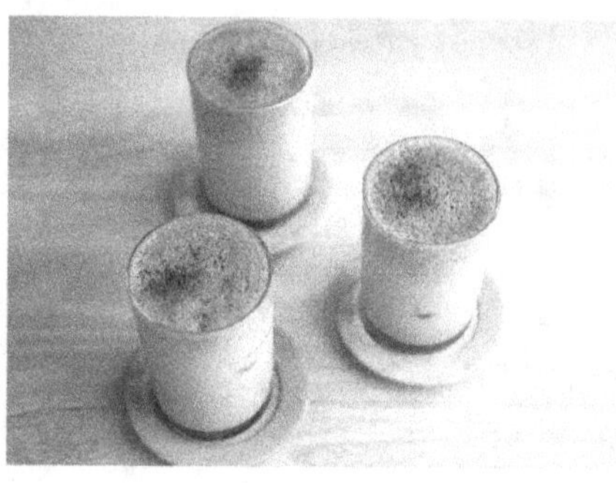

INGREDIENTS (for 2 servings)
Sweetened vanilla almond milk – 240 ml (Almond Breeze)
Matcha powder – 20 gr

INSTRUCTIONS
1. Pour almond milk in a shaker and add Matcha powder.
2. Shake well. Pour into 4 glasses.
Nutritional values (per 1 shot)
Carbs – 10 g, protein –1 g, fat – 2 g, energy – 55 kcal

90. Mango Banana Superfood Green Smoothie

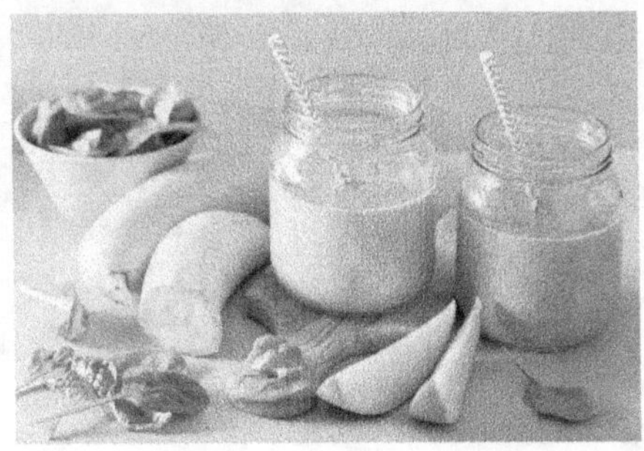

INGREDIENTS (for 2 servings)
Frozen banana – 1 piece
Baby spinach – 120 gr
Fresh mango – 2/3 cup
Raw hemp seeds – 50 gr
Unsweetened almond milk – 420 ml
Ice – 1 cup
Sweetener

INSTRUCTIONS
1. Dice mango, shell raw hemp seed (or buy shelled).
2. Blend all ingredients in a blender until smooth. Add sweetener if you like. Enjoy!
Nutritional values (per 1 smoothie (450 gr)
Carbs – 27 g, protein –5 g, fat – 6 g, energy – 173,5 kcal

91. Tropical Papaya Batido (fruit shake)

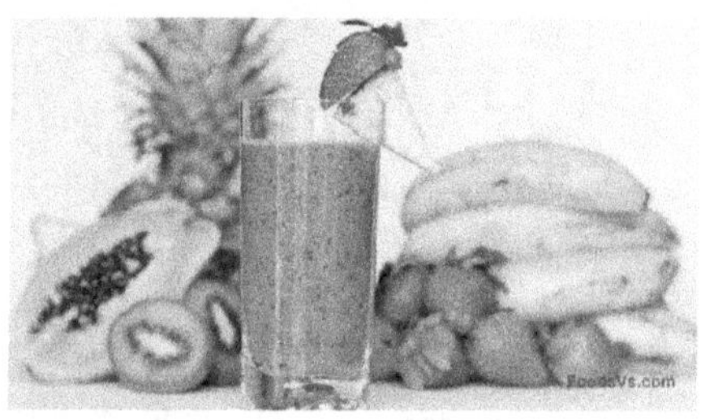

INGREDIENTS (for 2 servings)
Fresh papaya – 1 ½ cup
Banana – 1 piece
Orange juice – 480 ml
Crushed ice

INSTRUCTIONS
1. Squeeze fresh orange juice in a jug. Cut papaya.
2. Combine cutted papaya, banana and fresh squeezed orange juice in your blender.
3. Blend until smooth.
4. Serve with crushed ice!
Nutritional values (per 1 cup)
Carbs – 49 g, protein - 3 g, fat – 1 g, energy – 205 kcal

92. Strawberry And Rhubarb Compote Recipe

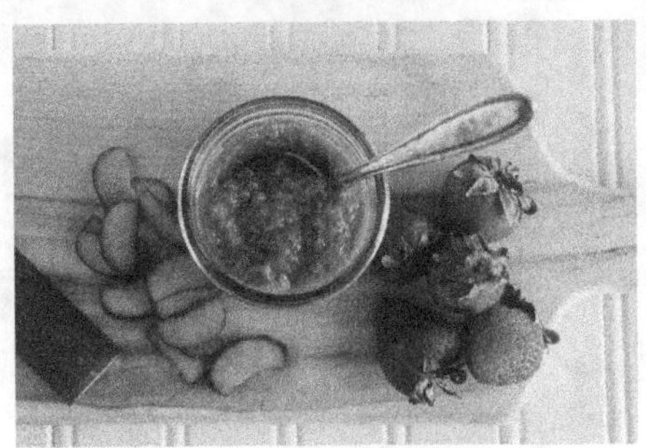

INGREDIENTS (for 4 servings)
Strawberry – 4 cups
Fresh rhubarb – 4 cups
Juice of one lemon
Water – 60 ml
Raw honey – 50 gr
Pinch of sea salt

INSTRUCTIONS
1. Chop strawberries and fresh rhubarb.
2. Put all the ingredients into a saucepan, add a pinch of salt.
3. Bring to a boil and simmer for half an hour until thickened.
4. Then blend until smooth.
5. Serve cool.
Nutritional values (per serving)
Carbs – 30 g, protein – 2 g, fat – 1 g

93. Mango and Strawberry Sorbet Recipe

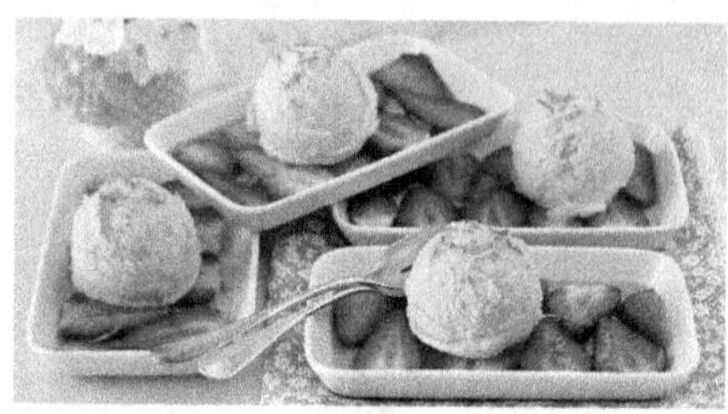

INGREDIENTS (for 4 servings)
Frozen mango – 4 cups
Frozen strawberries – 4 cups
 Water – 240 ml
Honey – 50 gr

INSTRUCTIONS
1. Combine 4 cups of frozen chopped mango, 4 cups of frozen chopped strawberries, 50 gr of honey and 240 ml of water in the blender.
2. Blend until smooth.
3. Pour in forms and freeze.
Nutritional values (per serving)
Carbs – 55 g, protein – 2 g, fat – 1 g

PALEO SOUPS

94. Turmeric Roasted Sweet Potato and Macadamia Soup

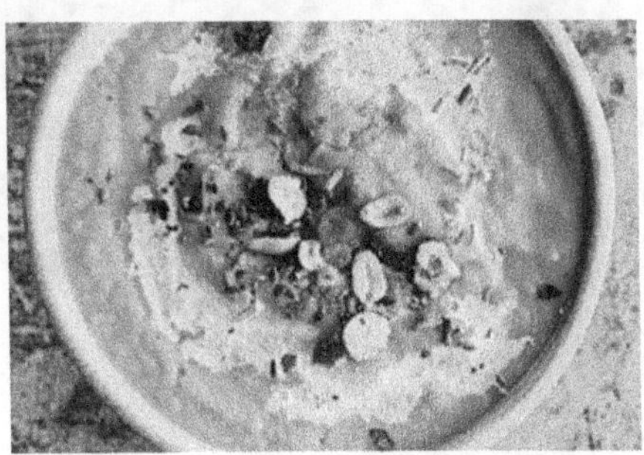

INGREDIENTS (for 9 servings)
Red onions – 2 pcs
Orange sweet potatoes – 1 kg
Extra-virgin olive oil – 15 ml
Vegetable broth – 1.9 l
Fresh ginger – 20 gr
Ground turmeric – 5 gr
Unsalted macadamias - 70 gr
Fresh lime wedges
Fresh cilantro – 50 gr
Pinch of cayenne pepper
Pinch of kosher sea salt
Chopped macadamias (Optional)

INSTRUCTIONS
1. In the very beginning heat the oven to 190 C. Then prepare vegetables: peel onion and cut into four parts, peel sweet potato and cut into chunks, chop fresh cilantro.
2. Use a parchment paper and line the baking sheet.
3. Roll onion parts and sweet potatoes chunks in oil and salt. Spread on the baking sheet. Roast in the preheated oven for an hour.
4. Take a large saucepan and pour in vegetable broth, add fresh minced ginger, ground turmeric, and a pinch of cayenne pepper. Bring to a boil. Cover and simmer 15 minutes.
5. Turn off the heat and add chopped macadamias. Leave the mixture for 10 minutes. Let nuts to soften a little.
6. Pour soup in the blender bowl and blend until smooth and creamy.

7. Pour soup into the saucepan again, flavor and warm.
8. Ladle this unbelievable tasty soup into portion dish. Drizzle with lime juice, chopped cilantro and chopped and macadamias.
9. Have you ever tried something similar???
Nutritional values (per 1 cup)
Carbs – 30,5 g, protein – 2,5 g, fat – 8 g, energy – 199 kcal

95. *Chunky Beef, Cabbage and Tomato Soup*

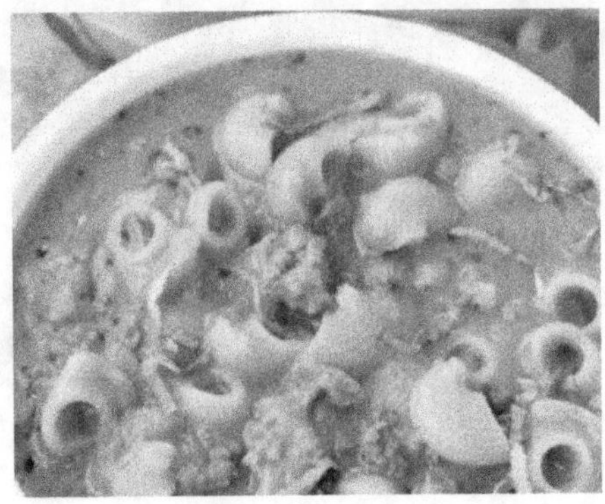

INGREDIENTS (for 7 servings – 11 cups)
Lean ground beef – 450 gr
Diced onion – 70 gr
Diced celery – 70 gr
Diced carrot – 70 gr
Diced tomatoes – 790 gr
Chopped green cabbage – 600 gr
Homemade beef stock – 950 ml
Bay leaves – 2 pcs
Kosher salt

INSTRUCTIONS
1. Heat the pan and add oil. Put salted ground beef and fry until golden brown (stir constantly and break the meat up to avoid big pieces).
2. After 5 minutes add diced onion, celery and carrot. Fry together for another 5 minutes.
3. Then add diced tomatoes, chopped green cabbage, and pour in homemade beef stock. Put bay leaves, cover the pan and cook 40 minutes.
4. After 40 minutes enjoy Chunky Beef, Cabbage and Tomato Soup!
Nutritional values (per 1,5 cup)
Carbs – 14 g, protein – 15,5 g, fat – 6 g, energy – 181 kcal

96. ROASTED BRUSSELS SPROUTS AND CAULIFLOWER SOUP

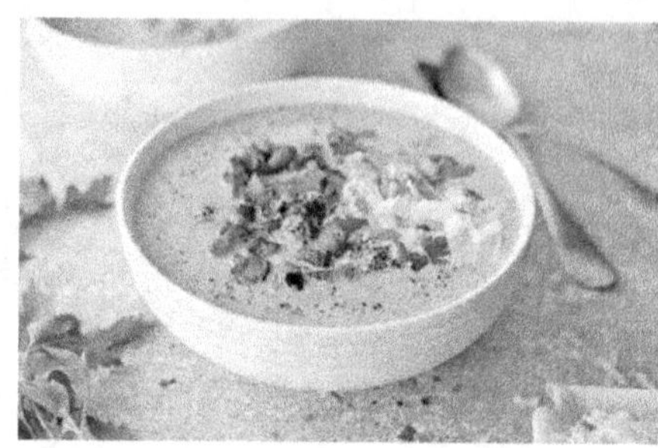

INGREDIENTS (for 4 servings)
Canola cooking spray
Cauliflower curds – 450 gr
Brussels sprouts – 450 gr
Olive oil – 30 ml
Butter – 10 gr
Chopped shallots – 50 gr
Vegetable broth – 850 ml
Kosher salt
Black pepper

INSTRUCTIONS
1. Heat your oven to 220 C.
2. Line baking tray with foil and grease with canola cooking spray. Divide cauliflower into curds and put each curd on the tray next to brussels sprouts. Spray with oil and bake for 25 minutes. Stir constantly.
3. When the cauliflower and brussels are baking, melt butter in a deep saucepan and add chopped shallots. Cook until soften. Pour in the vegetable broth and continue to simmer for 5 minutes more.
4. Take out the tray with roasted veggies and transfer them into the saucepan (rest 1 cup in the oven) and simmer for 2 minutes.
5. Transfer into the blender bowl and blend until smooth.
6. Pour soup in a bowl and top each portion with roasted vegetables and dust with fresh black pepper.
7. Enjoy immediately!
Nutritional values (per 1 cup + topping)
Carbs – 22 g, protein – 6,5 g, fat – 8 g, energy – 173 kcal

97. TURMERIC ROASTED CAULIFLOWER SOUP

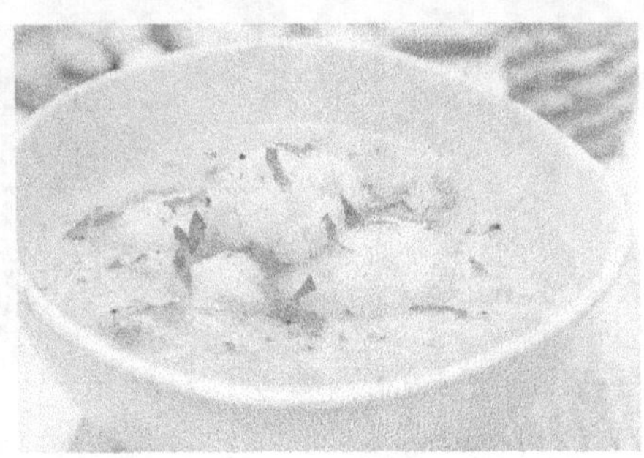

INGREDIENTS (for 4 servings)
Cauliflower curds – 6 heaping cups
Garlic bulbets – 3 pcs
Crushed red pepper flakes
Vegetable broth – 720 ml
Whole milk canned coconut milk – 60 ml
Chopped cilantro – 30 gr
Olive oil – 30 ml + 5 ml
Turmeric – 10 gr
Cumin – 10 gr
Kosher salt
Chopped onion

INSTRUCTIONS
1. Preheat the oven to 220°C. Smash garlic bulbets, divide cauliflower into curds.
2. Put cauliflower curds and smashed garlic in a separate bowl and sprinkle with olive oil. Toss all ingredients.
3. Take a small bowl and combine spices: turmeric, crushed red pepper flakes, cumin and salt. Dust over cauliflower curds and toss.
4. Spread flavored cauliflower on a baking sheet and bake until browned for half an hour. Reserve 1 cup.
5. After an hour, take a pot with oil and fry chopped onion. Pour in the broth and put reserved cauliflower, bring to a boil and simmer for 15 minutes.
6. Replace prepared cauliflower into the blender bowl and blend to a puree consistency. Try it and salt if necessary. Pour in coconut milk and stir.
7. Serve in separate plates, top with roasted cauliflower and chopped cilantro.
Nutritional values (per 1 1/8 cup)
Carbs – 14 g, protein – 4 g, fat – 10,5 g, energy – 159 kcal

98. SLOW COOKER BLISSFUL BUTTERNUT SQUASH SOUP

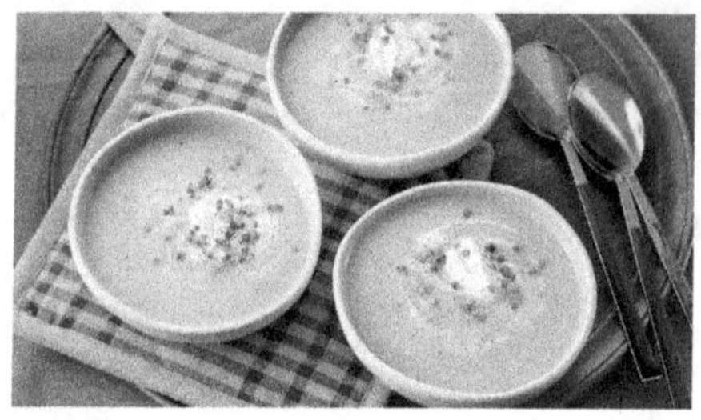

INGREDIENTS (for 4 servings)
Butternut squash – 450 gr
Kobacha squash – 450 gr
Shallot – 2 pcs
Vegetable broth – 500 ml
Coconut milk – 180 ml
A pinch of nutmeg

INSTRUCTIONS
1. Take a butternut squash, cut into halves and remove seeds. Do the same with kobacha squash. Quarter shallot.
2. Prepare a saucepan and put there halves of squash, shallots and pour vegetable broth.
3. Cook on low heat for 8 hours. Squash should be soft.
4. Remove the skin. Add coconut milk and a pinch of nutmeg. Stir well.
5. Blend this mass. Try it and add salt and pepper if necessary.
Nutritional values (per 1 ¼ cup)
Carbs – 35 g, protein –3 g, fat – 3 g, energy – 152 kcal

99. Tomato And Cucumber Gazpacho Recipe

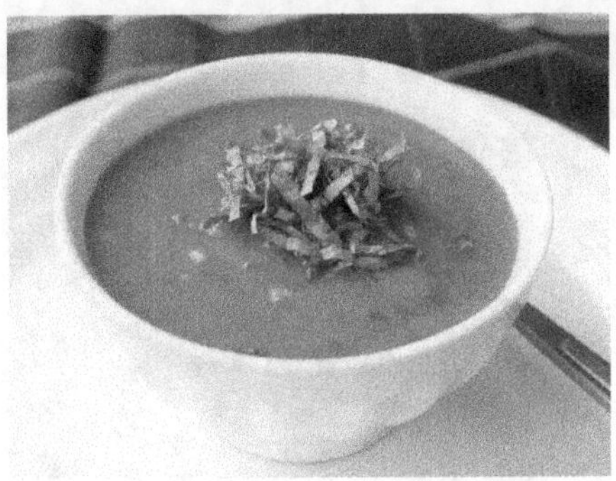

INGREDIENTS (for 4 servings)
Ripened tomatoes – 700 gr
Cucumber – 1 piece
Tomato juice – 1 l
Chopped red onion – ½
Fresh basil – ¼ cup
Fresh parsley – ¼ cup
Fresh cilantro – 50 gr
Garlic bulbets - 4pcs
Balsamic vinegar – 30 ml
Juice of one lime
Sea salt, ground black pepper

INSTRUCTIONS
1. Firstly, make preparations: peel and chop cucumber, then mince greens and garlic.
2. Bring a saucepan of water to a boil.
3. Make cuts at the bottom of each tomato. Put in a deep bowl.
4. Pour over the tomatoes boiling water. Let sit 2-3 minutes.
5. Remove tomatoes, peel them and dice.
6. Take a saucepan and pour tomato juice, lime juice, balsamic vinegar and the remaining water in it.
7. Add in minced greens and garlic; salt and pepper to taste.
8. Also add tomatoes and chopped cucumber. Stir well.
9. Chill before serving.
Nutritional values (per serving)
Carbs – 26 g, protein – 5 g, fat – 1 g

100. Mexican Chicken Soup Recipe

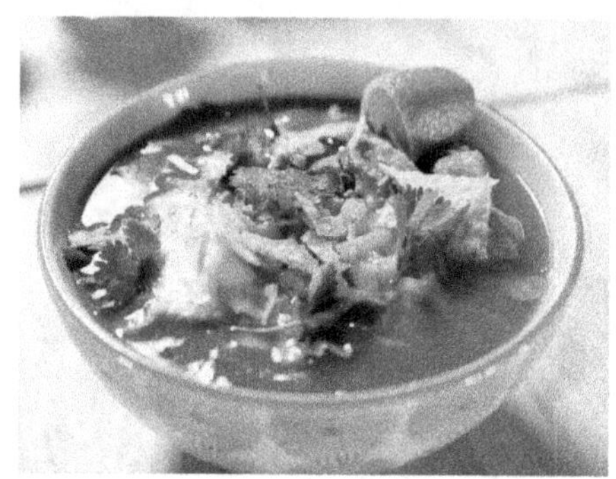

INGREDIENTS (for 4 servings)
Sweet potato – 1 piece
Paleo cooking fat - 50gr
Extra-virgin olive oil - 30ml
Onion-1/2
Garlic bulbets – 4 pcs
Ground cumin – 2 gr
Chicken stock – 1 l;
Roast chicken – ½
Cherry tomatoes – 1 cup
Fresh cilantro – 50 gr
Juice of half lime
Avocado – half
Sea salt, ground black pepper

INSTRUCTIONS
1. Make preparations: peel sweet potatoes and cut into cubes; slice onion; mince garlic; shred roast chicken; cut tomatoes in halves; chop cilantro and slice avocado.
2. Bring to a boil some water. Drop sweet potatoes cubes. Cook for 10 minutes. Drain the water and set aside.
3. Combine Paleo cooking fat and olive oil. Mix. Melt this fatty mixture in another saucepan.
4. Then add sliced onion and fry 5-7 min. Add minced garlic, ground cumin, salt and black pepper. Mix together and cook for a minute.
5. Pour in chicken stock and simmer for 2-3 min. Then put shredded chicken, halved tomatoes, lime juice, and prepared sweet potatoes. Drizzle with fresh cilantro. Once the soup comes to a boil, remove it immediately.
6. Let soup to sit for 5 minutes. Then serve this flavored soup. If desired, garnish with avocado slices.

Nutritional values (per serving)
Carbs – 13 g, protein – 70 g, fat – 26 g

Breakfast recipes

101. Bacon and egg Paradise

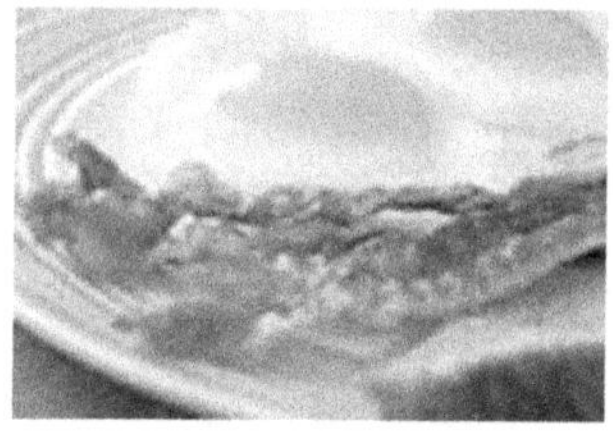

INGREDIENTS
3 - 6 eggs
3 slices of cut bacon
2 cups of spinach chopped
A bit of salt and pepper

INSTRUCTIONS
Heat your oven to 350F
Mix the eggs in a bowl
Cook the becon in a skillet
Add a spinach to this skillet and cook for 10 more minutes
Add eggs into this skillet and add a bit of salt and pepper.
Bake for 15 more minutes

102. Perfect Paleo Pancakes (nut-free)

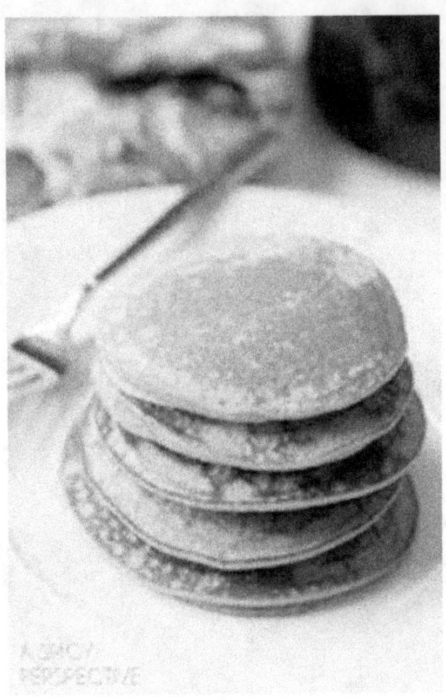

INGREDIENTS
4 Eggs
Half of a cup of coconut flour
1table spoon of honey
1 table spoon of vinegar
a half of a spoon of baking soda
a bit of a salt
1 table spoon of vanilla

INSTRUCTIONS
Put all the dry pancake ingredients in a bowl. Whip in all the liquid ingredients (do not add the coconut milk).
Gradually add the coconut milk. You will need to add as much coconut milk as you need until you see the preferable consistency.
Preheat a consistency and coat with grease with coconut oil.
Pour a spoon of a pancake batter onto the griddle. Make the pancakes about 3-4 inches in diameter as it will be easier to operate them. Bake for 2-3 minutes, then turn them on another side for an additional 1-2 minutes.
Take away from a pan and serve with your chosen syrup.

Enjoy your breakfast.

103. Paleo Blueberry Muffin

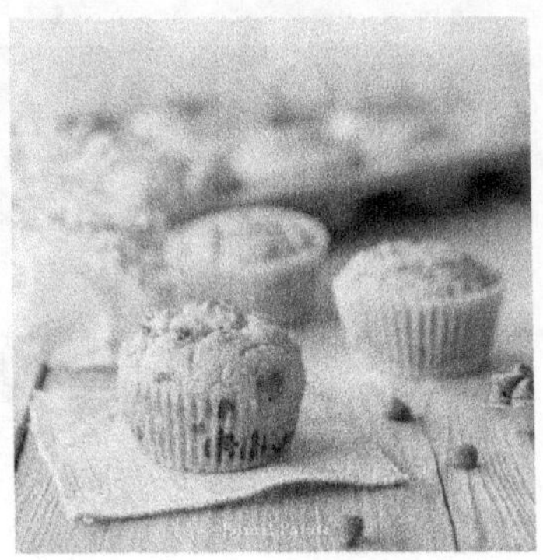

INGREDIENTS
1 cup of almond flour
A bit of soda
A bit of salt on your taste
1 egg
2 tbsp of honey
A half of a cup of fresh blueberries
A half of a cup of coconut milk
2 tbsp of coconut oil

INSTRUCTIONS
1. Heat the oven to 350°F.
2. Mix all together salt, baking soda and almond flour
3. Whip all together the honey, coconut milk, coconut oil, and egg.
4. Then mix the wet and the dry ingredients together, but not that much.
5. Add blueberries into the dough.
6. Add the prepared dough into the muffin tin and bake
7. Bake until a toothpick inserted into the center comes out clean, about 20-25 minutes
8. Set pan over a wire rack to cool. Wait until muffins are completely cool before removing from the paper liners.

Recipe makes 6 muffins. Store in an airtight container in the refrigerator.

104. Paleo Breakfast: Baked Eggs in Ham Cups

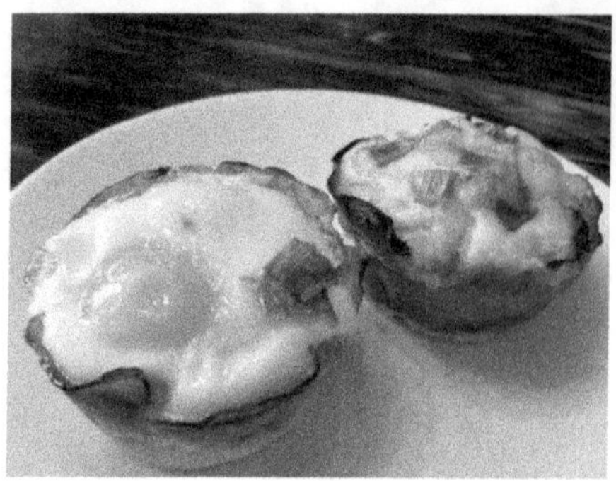

INGREDIENTS
Eggs
Ham or Turkey

INSTRUCTIONS
1. Heat the oven to 400°F.
2. Grease your muffin pan.
3. Slice the ham and put it into the muffin cup, one or two slices is enough for each cup.
4. You can scramble your eggs or even whip them or you can just put the whole egg into the muffin cup. (Optional) If you do wish to make scrambled eggs you can also add there different ingredients, like mushrooms, onion, different greens and spinach.
5. Preheat the oven ti 400°F , put the muffin pan in to the oven and bake for 15 – 20 more minutes

105. Avocado & Bacon Muffins

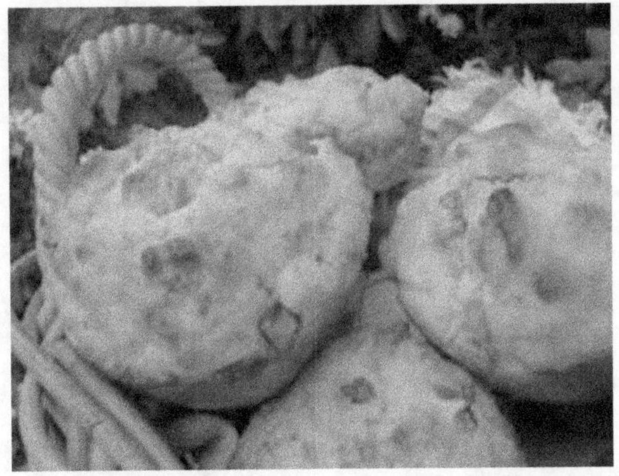

INGREDIENTS
1 onion
4 eggs
6 -7 slices of bacon
2 cups avocado
one and a half of a cup of coconut flour
a half of a tea spoon of baking soda
salt & pepper
1 cup of coconut milk

INSTRUCTIONS
1. Heat the oven to 175 degrees Celsius (350F)
2. Grease 12 muffin pans with oil. (melt it before)
3. Finely chop onion and bacon.
4. Brown in a fry pan.
5. Mix the avocado and eggs very good.
6. Stir in the milk.
7. Add coconut flour, salt, pepper and baking soda and stir it all well
8. Fold through three quarters of the cooked bacon and onion mixture.
9. Put this into the muffin pans.

10. Put on the top bacon and onion.
11. Bake in the oven for approximately 20 25 minutes.
12. Cool before taking the muffins out. 13. Enjoy your breakfast.

LUNCH RECIPES

106. Super Paleo Chinese Chicken Salad

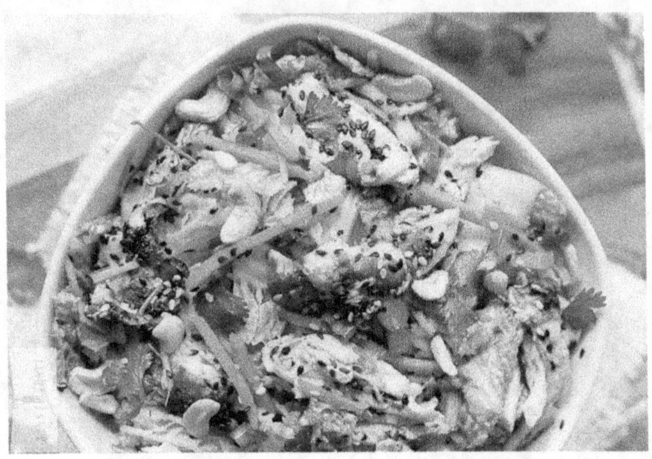

INGREDIENTS

1 carrot

1 large Napa Cabbage, it is necessary to chop it into slices.

1 chicken, sliced into thin peaces.

A half of a cup chopped cilantro

2 tablespoons of black sesame seeds and 2 table spoons of white sesame seeds

1/4 cup of gluten free soy sauce, I prefer Tamari.

1/4 cup white wine vinegar

3 table spoons of a minced ginger

3 table spoons of olive oil

1 table spoon of toasted sesame oil

1 table spoon of Spicy Chili Oil

Some sea salt on your taste

Some chopped green onions

INSTRUCTIONS

In a small bowl with lid add tamari sauce, vinegar, olive oil, hoisin sauce, toasted sesame oil, chili oil, sriracha, minced ginger, sea salt and chopped green onions. Shake it all together. Set aside. Then add, chopped cabbage, sliced carrot, cilantro, sesame seeds, cashews, sliced chicken, and dressing into a large plastic bowl, shake until well enough. Add more dressing if needed.

107. Spicy Tuna and Tomato

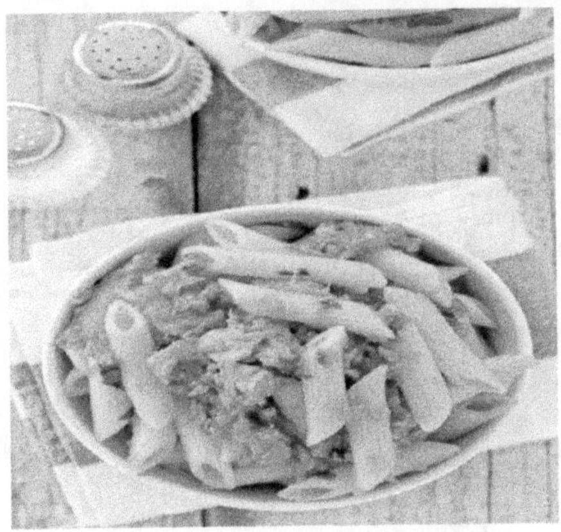

INGREDIENTS

1 cup of tuna

1 red onion, chopped

1 small red chilli, chopped as well

1 peace of garlic

1 egg

2 Tbsp of tomato paste

1 Tbsp of coconut flour

Salt and pepper on your taste

You can also add:

Lettuce

Avocado

Extra chilli, if you wish it to be hot

INSTRUCTIONS

1 – Pre-heat your oven to 350'F

2 – Put a parchment paper on a baking tray and set aside for now.

3 – Put all the burger ingredients into a bowl and stir all them well

4. Make with your hands bolls using this tuna mixture. Place all of them into the baking sheet

5 – Place in the oven and cook approximately for 5-10 mins, until they are cooked enough.

6 – To serve, place these cute balls on a lettuce leaf (or 2) put some fresh sliced avocado on top, and sprinkle over some fresh coriander and some slices of chilli.

Enjoy your meal!

108. Cucumber and Tomato Salad

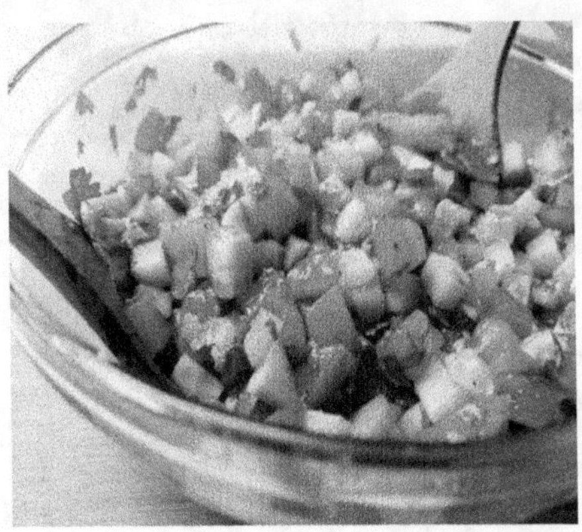

INGREDIENTS

one clove Garlic

one cup of Olives

one tablespoon of fresh Basil, (it is necessary to slice it very thin)

one table spoon of Fresh Oregano, (it is necessary to chop it)

two cups of Cucumber, sliced or chopped.

Two cups of Grape Tomatoes

Two table spoons of Balsamic Vinegar

Two table spoons of Extra Virgin Olive Oil

One table spoon of Black Pepper

INSTRUCTIONS

1. Rinse, then slice or chop your cucumbers.
2. Rinse grape tomatoes, cut them in half.
3. Thinly slice basil, cut oregano, mince garlic.
4. Mix everything with the kalamata olives in a bowl, sprinkle with olive oil and balsamic vinegar, and add a bit of black pepper.

109. Chicken and avocado Lettuce Wraps

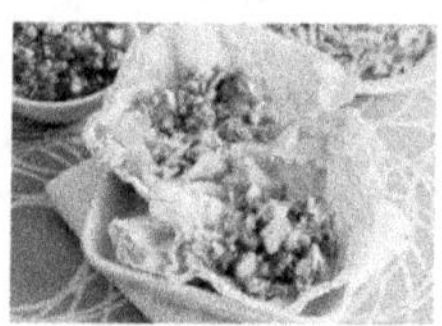

INGREDIENTS

One cup cooked and sliced Chicken, Boneless Breasts

One and a half cup of mashed avocado, peel the coat before mashing.

one tbsp. of juice Lemon

one tbsp. of juice Lime

two tbsp. of Yogurt

two tbsp of choped Cilantro

Salt on your taste

Black Pepper on your taste

Serving Day Ingredients

One cup of grape tomatoes

INSTRUCTIONS

1. Chop chicken breast
2. Mash avocado, lemon juice, lime juice, and yogurt in a bowl and stir well, until it becomes creamy!
3. Add salt, pepper and cilantro to the chopped chicken, according to your taste.
4. Spoon into lettuce wraps, put tomatoes on top, and serve.

110. Swett Potato

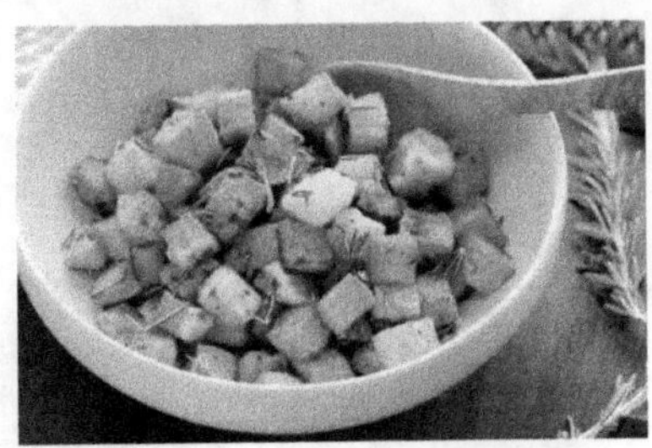

INGREDIENTS

2 Medium sweet potatoes chopped into small cubes
3 tbsp of coconut oil
Sea salt

INSTRUCTIONS

1. Boil water in a medium pot
2. Chop sweet potato into cubes
3. Put the sweet potato into the boiling water for around five minutes and take It away when it becomes slightly softened.
4. Drain and dry the sweet potatoes
5. Heat up the coconut oil in the large skillet, make the heat medium.
6. Toss in the sweet potatoes cubes and let them cook well for approximately six or seven minutes. Continue doing it until they are nice and brown. Sprinkle with sea salt according to your taste. Your sweet potatoes will be yummy, crispy and goldy brown if you let them cook well enough.

ENJOY YOUR MEAL!

DINNER RECIPES

111.Paleo Pizza Soup

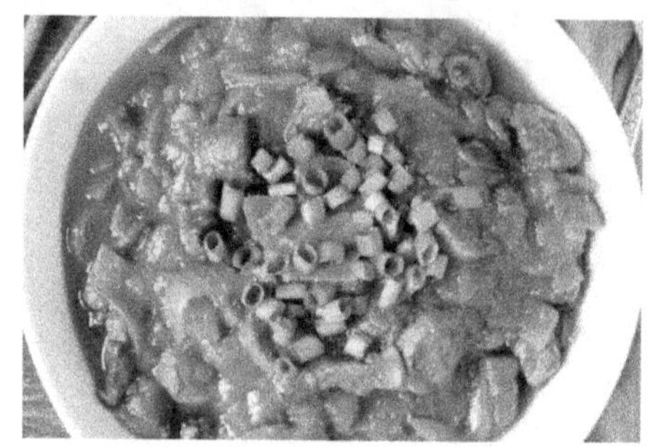

INGREDIENTS

10-12 chicken sausage, slice them

4 – 5 uncured pepperoni,

5-7 roasted tomatoes

1 medium size onion,

10-15 mushrooms, slice them

1 can of black olives, slice them

1 tbsp of dried oregano

1 tsp of garlic powder

Salt to taste

INSTRUCTIONS

1. Put the sausage, pepperoni, marinara, tomatoes, onion, mushrooms, olives, oregano, garlic powder, and salt into the pan
2. Cook for about 30 minutes. It is considered to be ready when onions and mushrooms have softened.
3. Add more salt if needed.
4. Serve hot.
5. Enjoy this delicious meal.

112. Quick and Easy Fish Curry

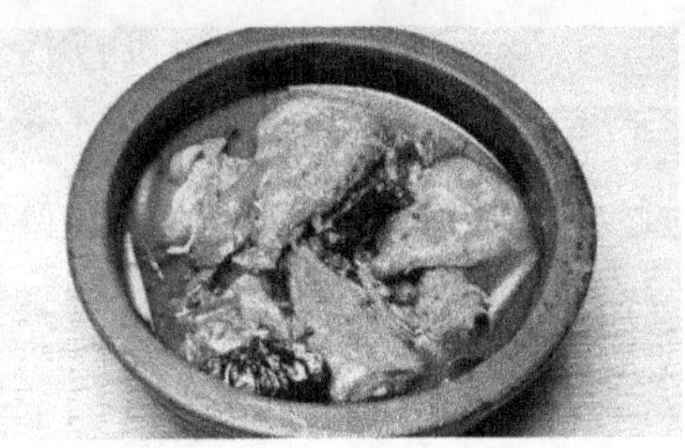

INGREDIENTS

2 Tbsp of coconut oil

1 onion,

3 cloves of garlic, chopped or mashed

2 Tbsp of ginger

2 tsp of curry powder

10 - 15 curry leaves

400ml of coconut milk

2 tomatoes, chopp them

Sea salt on your taste

600g of white fish, cut into peaces

Juice of a lime on your taste

Large handful leaves of coriander

INSTRUCTIONS

1. Melt the coconut oil in the pan.
2. Add sliced onion there and make it brown
3. Than add the garlic and ginger and cook for approximately one minute.
4. Add the turmeric, curry leaves and do not forget about the curry powder.
5. Continue to cook during one minute, then gradually stir in the coconut milk.
6. Simmer it.
7. Add the chopped tomato and simmer for additional five minutes until the tomato become soft.
8. Add the fish, add some salt on your taste and wait until the fish is cooked.
9. Add coriander and lime juice and stir it all well.
10. It is a very delicious with rice

113. Paleo Pineapple Fried Rice

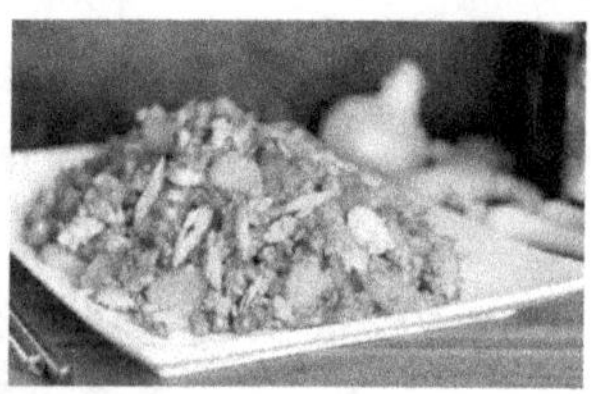

INGREDIENTS
Three table spoons of avocado oil
two cups of fresh pineapple, cut for the slices
one red bell pepper
four small carrots
two cloves garlic, minced
a bit of green onions, thinly sliced
four eggs

Sauce:
¼ cup coconut aminos
2 tsp of chili paste

As a final step:
one cup of roasted cashew pieces
Sea salt on your taste

INSTRUCTIONS
1. Prepare all your ingredients, wash and cut them
2. Take away the core with its seeds from the bell pepper and cut it thoroughly.
3. Peel the carrots and cut it into cubes.
4. Grate the cauliflower.
5. Crack the eggs into a plastic bowl and mix them with the fork or whatever.
6. Put together the coconut aminos and chili paste in a bowl and set it aside.
7. After you have prepared everything, preheat your pan
8. Add one tbsp of the avocado oil to the frying pan and also add the pineapple chunks to create the tasty and caramelized edges. Then take away the pineapples and put it into the separate bowl, until you prepare the rice. After add the green onions and cauliflower. It is necessary to cook it for about several minutes to make the cauliflower soft.
9. Then add all the veggies into the pan; pepper, garlic, carrots and make them crispy.

10. Add the sauce to the pan and let it to prepare for several more minutes until the sauce is gone and mix everything well.
11. Take away the fried rice from the heat and join it to cashews and caramelized pineapple. Add some sea salt if necessary. It tastes simply amazing both hot and taken from the refrigerator.

114. Paleo Mini Meatloaves

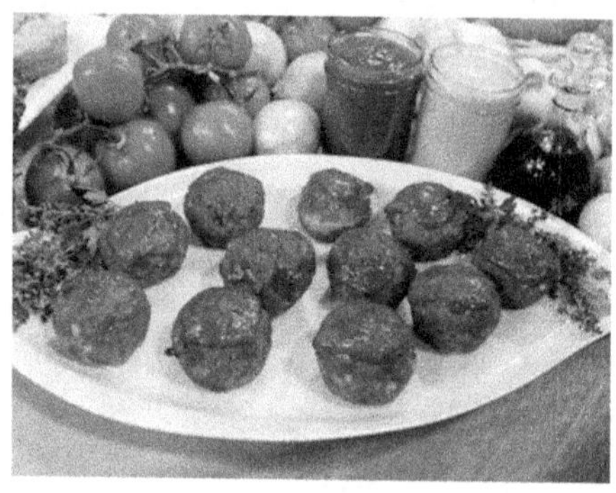

INGREDIENTS

two pounds of meat – it is better to mix beef with pork or veal

chopped spinach, the amount on your preference

one or two teaspoons oil

one medium onion,

ten - fifteen mushrooms, finely diced

two grated carrots,

four eggs,

1/3 cup coconut flour

two tsp of salt

two tsp of pepper

two tsp of onion powder

one tsp of garlic powder

one tsp of dried thyme and a bit of grated nutmeg.

INSTRUCTIONS

1. Preheat oven to 375 degrees F
2. Prepare spinach and set aside.
3. Preheat a pan add the oil and add there onions, mushrooms. Cook everything until the onion become translucent and some water is gone. Than you can set this pan aside. Place the ground meat in a large bowl, add the spinach, carrots, mushroom/onion mixture, beaten eggs, coconut flour and all the spices. Mix everything, but not that much, just to make all the ingredients well – organized.
4. Add this mixture into muffin tins. It is better to grease the tins.
5. Cook for 20-25 minutes until total preparation.

6. This dish is better to serve hot.

115. Stuffed Baby Sweet Peppers

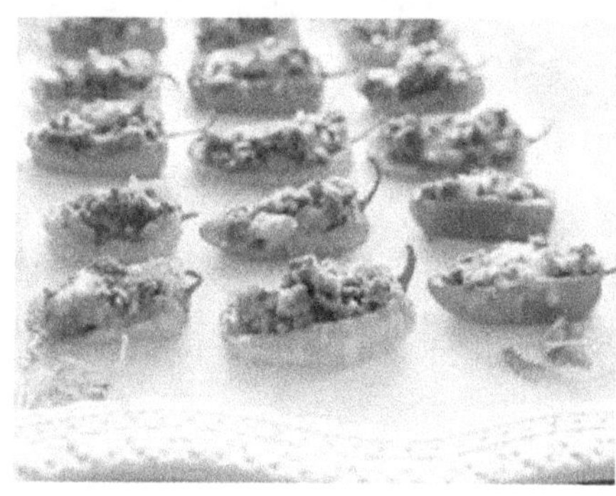

INGREDIENTS

Fifteen - twenty mini sweet peppers
Six ounces of goat cheese
A half of a cup of ricotta cheese
One tea spoon of garlic powder
A bit of pepper powder
Salt to your taste

INSTRUCTIONS

1. Preheat oven to 375F. Lean baking sheet with foil.
2. Wash the peppers and cut in half lengthwise. Remove all the seeds
3. Than mash together the goat cheese, the ricotta, and the seasonings well.
4. Snip the corner off of a small ziploc bag and put cheese mixture into this bag. Squeeze the bag and pipe the cheese into the pepper halves.
5. Put the peppers on the baking sheet and cook it for about 5-6 minutes until nicely browned. It is possible to prepare this delicious thing on the grill as well.
6. Enjoy!

Some more Paleo Recipes

116. Creamy Lemon Basil Spaghetti Squash

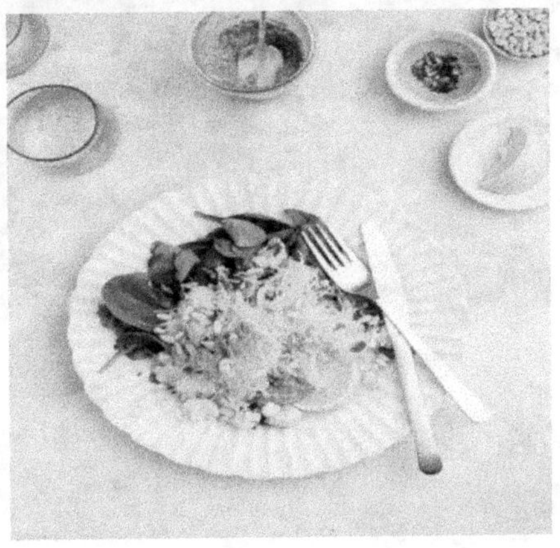

INGREDIENTS
One Avocado (a half of a cup mashed)
six garlic cloves
one cup fresh basil leaves
one tbsp lemon zest
one third of a cup lemon juice
 two tbsp. of olive oil

INSTRUCTIONS
if you wish you can add cayenne pepper on your taste
 a half of tsp black pepper
a sea salt on your taste

117. Spaghetti Squash

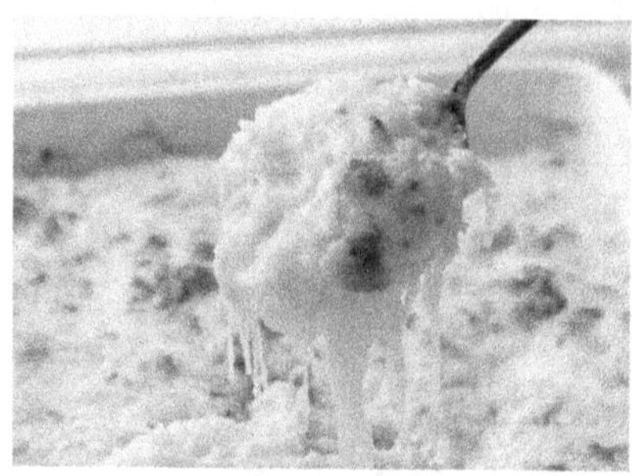

INGREDIENTS
two tsp olive oil
three cups spaghetti squash, cooked
one cup of chopped kale
10-15 cherry tomatoes
A half of tsp black pepper
sea salt on your taste

INSTRUCTIONS
1. Mix all the sauce ingredients into blender. Puree them thoroughly
2. Heat the pan and add the olive oil. When the oil is hot add the tomatoes and sauté about two minutes.
3. Add the other ingredients and sauté approximately five minutes. Add about a half of a cup of the sauce and mix thoroughly.
4. Bon appetite!!!

118. Butternut Squash Risotto

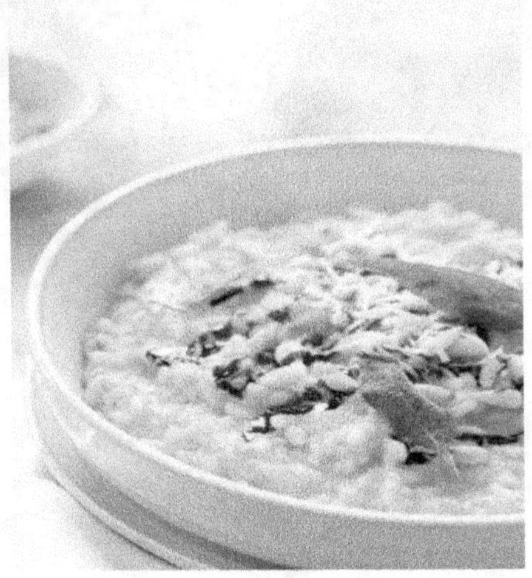

INGREDIENTS

1½ pounds butternut squash, peeled and cubed (about 4 cups)

1 tablespoon solid cooking fat

½ yellow onion, chopped

1 cup mushrooms, chopped

3 cloves garlic, minced

¼ cup sage, minced

½ teaspoon sea salt

1 teaspoon apple cider vinegar

¾ cup bone broth

INSTRUCTIONS

1. Place half of the chopped butternut squash into a food processor and pulse for 20 seconds, until the squash is the consistency of rice. Don't over process here!

2. Heat the solid cooking fat in the bottom of a large skillet or heavy-bottomed pot on medium heat. When the fat has melted and the pan is hot, add the onions and mushrooms. Cook, stirring, until the onions are translucent, about 5 minutes. Add the garlic, sage, and sea salt, and cook for another 2 minutes, just until fragrant.

3. Add the apple cider vinegar and scrape away anything that has stuck to the bottom of the pan. Add the processed squash and bone broth to the pan, stirring to incorporate. Cook for 12-15 minutes on medium heat uncovered, stirring occasionally, until the liquid has absorbed and the squash is fully cooked.

119. Coconut Crusted Chicken Salad

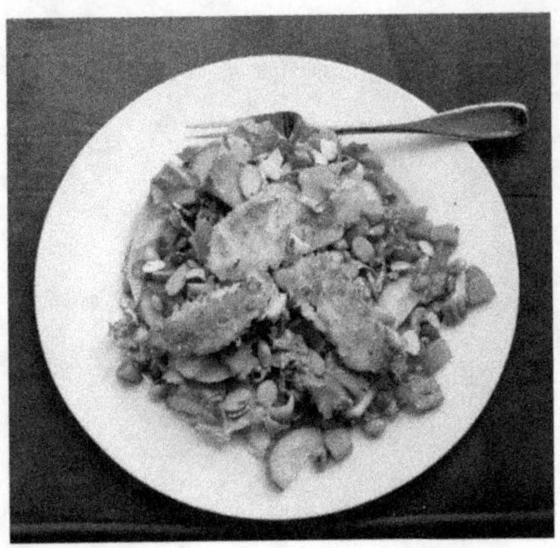

INGREDIENTS

2 tbsp Coconut flour

2 tbsp Unsweetened flaked coconut

2 Chicken fillets

1 Egg (beaten)

2 cups Spring mix salad greens

3 tbsp Apple cider vinegar

1 tsp Honey

3 tbsp olive oil

2 tbsp Coconut oil

Salt and pepper (to taste)

INSTRUCTIONS

1. Create a breading/dredging station with three plates or shallow bowls.
2. Add the coconut flour to one, the the egg to the second plate and the flaked coconut to the third.
3. Heat the coconut oil in a skillet over medium-high heat.
4. Dredge each chicken fillet in the coconut flour first, followed by the egg, coating each evenly. Then the flaked coconut. Be sure the fillet is coated well.
5. Place each fillet into the hot skillet. Cook on each side, about 5 minutes. Until the chicken is golden in color and cooked through.
6. Add the apple cider vinegar and honey to a bowl. Whisk to combine. Continue to whisk while drizzling in the olive oil until well combined and becomes creamy. Season with salt and pepper.

7. Place the spring mix in a mixing bowl. Drizzle the dressing over and toss to coat. Reserve ½ to serving. Plate the spring mix evenly then serve the chicken on top. Serve with additional dressing on the side. Season with salt and pepper, to taste.

120. Paleo Crock Pot Cashew Chicken

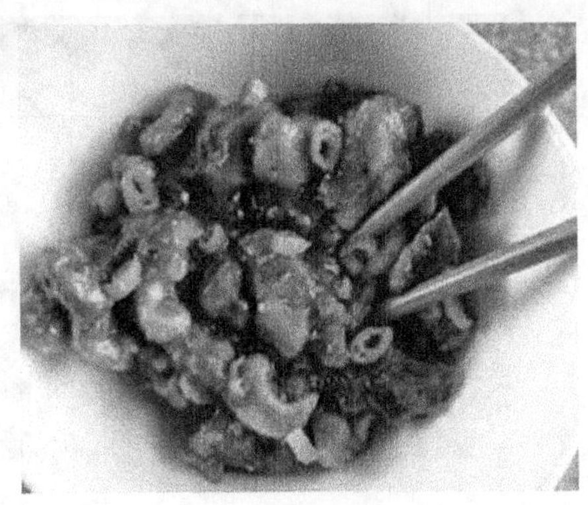

INGREDIENTS
1/4 cup arrowroot starch
1/2 tsp. black pepper
2 lbs. chicken thighs, cut into bite-size pieces
1 tbs. coconut oil
3 tbs. coconut aminos
2 tbs. rice wine vinegar
2 tbs. organic ketchup (tomato paste would work also)
1/2-1 tbs. palm sugar
2 minced garlic cloves
1/2 tsp. minced fresh ginger
1/4-1/2 red pepper flakes
1/2 cup raw cashews

INSTRUCTIONS
Place starch and black pepper in a large Ziploc bag. Add chicken pieces and seal; toss to thoroughly coat meat. Melt coconut oil in a large skillet or wok. Add chicken and cook for about 5 minutes until brown on all sides. Remove and add to crock pot.
Mix coconut aminos through red pepper flakes in a small bowl. Pour mixture over chicken and toss to coat. Put lid on crock pot and cook on low for 3-4 hours.
Stir cashews into chicken and sauce before serving.

121. Fried Cabbage with Bacon, Onion, and Garlic

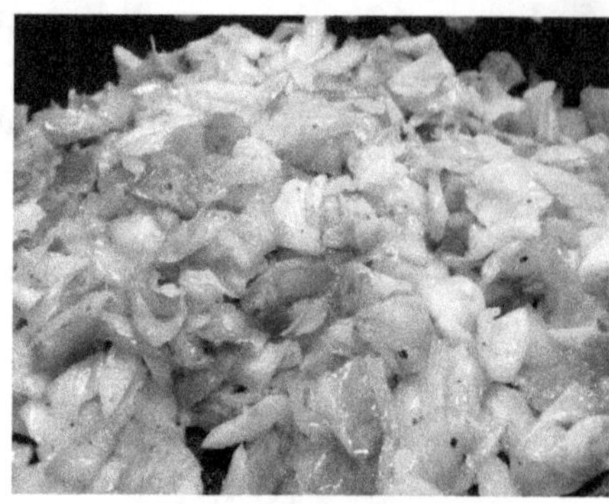

INGREDIENTS

Six slices of chopped becon
one large onion
two cloves of garlic
One cabbage
Salt on your taste
Pepper on your taste
A half of a teaspoon of onion powder
A half of a tea spoon of garlic powder

INSTRUCTIONS

Put the bacon in a large stockpot and cook it until it becomes crispy. It should take you about ten minutes. Add the garlic and onion. cook until the onion caramelizes; about ten minutes. Then Stir in the cabbage and continue to cook and stir for another 10 minutes. Add salt, pepper, onion powder, paprika and garlic powder. After all simmer for about 30 minutes more.

122. Roasted Tasty Vegetable Medley

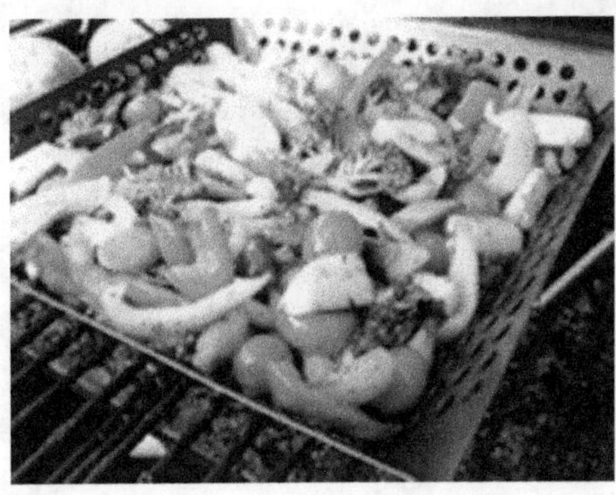

INGREDIENTS

2 tbsp olive oil

One yam, peeled and cut into pieces.

One parsnip, peeled and cut into pieces.

One carrot

One zucchini, cut into pieces

One bunch of a fresh asparagus, also cut into pieces

Two cloves of a minced garlic

Fresh basil, on your taste

Pepper on your taste

INSTRUCTIONS

1. Heat the oven and grease the baking sheet with olive oil.
2. Put the yams, parsnips, and carrots onto the baking sheets. Bake in the oven for 30 minutes, after put the zucchini and asparagus, and sprinkle with the 1 tablespoon of olive oil. Proceed baking until all of the vegetables are cooked, about 30 minutes more. Then remove from the oven, and allow to cool.
3. Toss the roasted peppers with the garlic, basil, salt, and pepper in a large bowl. Add the roasted vegetables, and mix everything well.

123. Delicious Beet Greens

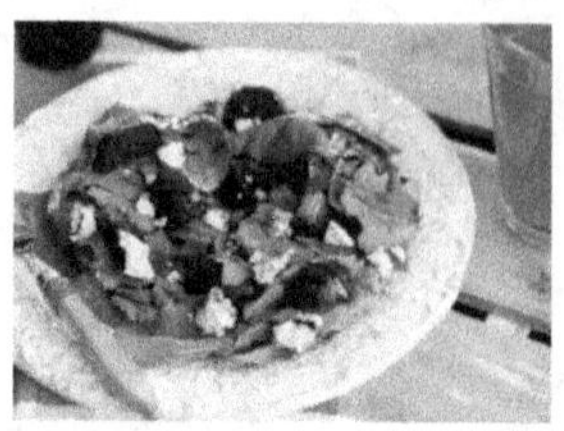

INGREDIENTS

Two bunches beet greens
One table spoon of olive oil
Two cloves of garlic minced
Red pepper on your taste
Salt and pepper on your taste
Two lemons, cut into four slices

INSTRUCTIONS

1. Put water into a pot let it to boil and salt it. Add the beet greens and cook them until they become tender. It will take you about two minutes. Drain beet greens then immerse with the ice water.
2. Bring a large pot of lightly salted water to a boil. Add the beet greens, and cook uncovered until tender, about 2 minutes. Drain in a colander, then immediately immerse in ice water for several minutes. Then chop the greens.
3. Heat the olive oil. Stir in the garlic and red pepper; cook and stir for one minute. Add salt and pepper. Cook until greens are hot; serve with lemon.

Thank You!

I am very happy that you have chosen this book and it's been a real pleasure writing it for you. My aim is to help as many readers as possible. So many of us are able to take new knowledge and use it to our lives with really useful and long lasting consequences and it is my desire that you have been able to take value from the information I have written.

Thank you for beeing with me during this book and for reading it through to the end. I really hope that you have enjoyed the information and that's why I appreciate your thoughts on my material so much. If you could take a couple of minutes to write a feedback, your views will help me to create more material that you find beneficial.

Thanks again for your attention. I really look forward to reading your review.

Stay Healthy!

www.ingramcontent.com/pod-product-compliance
Lightning Source LLC
Chambersburg PA
CBHW080846260726
48660CB00009B/3219